Praise for
Bursting with Energy

"Dr. Shallenberger's book is bursting with compelling new insights into health and longevity."

—Wendy Whitworth, Executive Producer, *Larry King Live*

"Bursting with Energy is also bursting with practical information for the lay person and for the busy practitioner. With mathematical precision, this book adds up to a true set of rules for health and healthy living. Some books you buy and never read; this one you will read and reread for the easy flow of ideas, the proven guidelines for staying young, and the clear answers about how and why they work."

—Richard Kunin, M.D., author of *Mega-Nutrition*

"Well-written and thorough. This innovative book provides very practical methods for increasing your energy production at any age."

—Hyla Cass, M.D., author of *All About Herbs*,
Supplement Your Prescription, and other popular health books

"This book provides dramatic information on stuffing yourself with oxygen, the single greatest preventer of chronic and degenerative disease."

—Robert Rowen, M.D., Editor-in-Chief,
Second Opinion Newsletter

BURSTING WITH ENERGY

THE BREAKTHROUGH METHOD TO RENEW YOUTHFUL ENERGY AND RESTORE HEALTH

FRANK SHALLENBERGER, M.D., H.M.D.

Foreword by Jonathan Wright, M.D.

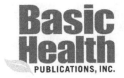

Basic
Health
PUBLICATIONS, INC.

The information contained in this book is based upon the research and personal and professional experiences of the author. It is not intended as a substitute for consulting with your physician or other healthcare provider. Any attempt to diagnose and treat an illness should be done under the direction of a healthcare professional.

The publisher does not advocate the use of any particular healthcare protocol but believes the information in this book should be available to the public. The publisher and author are not responsible for any adverse effects or consequences resulting from the use of the suggestions, preparations, or procedures discussed in this book. Should the reader have any questions concerning the appropriateness of any procedures or preparation mentioned, the author and the publisher strongly suggest consulting a professional healthcare advisor.

Basic Health Publications, Inc.
28812 Top of the World Drive
Laguna Beach, CA 92651
949-715-7327 • www.basichealthpub.com

Library of Congress Cataloging-in-Publication Data
Shallenberger, Frank.
    Bursting with energy / Frank Shallenberger ; foreword by Jonathan Wright. — 2nd ed.
        p. cm.
    Includes bibliographical references and index.
    ISBN 978-1-59120-127-4
    1. Longevity. 2. Energy metabolism. 3. Fatigue. I. Title.

    RA776.75.S455   2007
    613—dc22

                                                        2007015618

Editor: Roberta W. Waddell
Typesetting/Book design: Gary A. Rosenberg
Cover design: Mike Stromberg

Printed in the United States of America

10   9   8   7   6   5   4   3   2   1

Contents

Appendices

*To my patients, the most wonderful group of people
a doctor could ever hope to serve.*

You have allowed me to practice on you for years.

You have given your trust and often bared your souls.

*You have faced the uncertainty of sickness and
the certainty of death with great strength and courage.*

*You have given me support when I needed it most,
and have taught me more about life and medicine
than all my medical books and training.*

*In you, I have often been privileged to see the beauty
and magnificence that humans are capable of.
I feel humbled and honored in your presence.*

*This book is also dedicated to my wife and children,
who have had to endure everything from coffee enemas
to soyburgers as part of my particular search for truth.*

Foreword

Natural healthcare and natural medicine really aren't hard. We just need to read our human blueprints and follow them. It's just common sense. We do this if we're trying to maintain or repair anything else. Find the original plans, the original specifications, and work with or duplicate them. To repair broken equipment, we find parts identical to the damaged ones, put them in place just as the original plan specifies, and the equipment works again. No big deal. Maintenance is done like this all the time, everywhere.

Unless you're a doctor.

If you're a doctor, you try to repair humans with parts never, ever found in the original blueprints. Where the human biochemical plan calls for a protein or an amino acid, you use a patent medicine (pharmaceutical drug). Where the plan specifies a vitamin, you use a patent medicine. Where the plan calls for a combination of essential fatty acids, zinc, and vitamin A, you use . . . a patent medicine.

Is it any wonder that more than 100,000 people in the USA reportedly die of adverse reactions to patent medicines? The real surprise is that patent medicines do any good at all, since they're simply not part of our original design.

It's as if an entire country's mechanics insisted on fixing automobiles with airplane parts. It wouldn't make any sense. Customers would be screaming at them to follow the original plan. Use automobile parts for automobiles, and never mind whether the Federal Automobile Administration approves or not, the customers would demand. It's just common sense.

Dr. Frank Shallenberger is a very unusual doctor. He follows the original human blueprint, even though he, too, was educated to use parts that have never, ever been part of the blueprint of human malfunction repair. For several years, he recommended patent medicines as he'd been taught in medical school. After observing that using airplane parts to fix automobiles didn't work, he did something very unusual (for a doctor); he decided to figure out for himself what would really work, and in this book, he shares his discoveries with us.

Dr. Shallenberger went back to basic principles. He decided to apply the factors that have supported human life for literally hundreds of thousands of years (not one of them a patent medicine) and . . . they *worked*.

Water

Rest

Sunlight

Food (real food, please)

Exercise

Breathing (healthfully)

Simple things, but things we all need to *re*learn in the twenty-first century. Come to think of it, humans have needed to relearn them for several centuries, since our way of life has strayed so far from that of original humanity.

But Dr. Shallenberger doesn't expect or want us to live as original, primitive humans. He blends the factors that have helped keep humans healthy over thousands of generations with real improvements that modern scientific knowledge has brought to healthcare:

Supplements (no one ever knew about vitamins a century ago);

Natural (not synthetic or horse) hormone replacement;

An advanced knowledge of human biochemistry that allows for a much more accurate diagnosis and treatment.

In addition, he's put together a testing system that, logically enough, measures your body's basic air intake and output to gauge how efficiently your body works. Even though his system is quite innovative, it's just common sense (again). It's just like testing automobile exhaust to determine how efficiently the engine works. Even better, if a malfunction is found, he can tell us how to fix it.

Please don't think I am unappreciative of some of the tremendous advances made in medicine over the last century. Dr Shallenberger and I agree that if you get run over by a truck, it doesn't matter whether the truck carried whole, natural organic food or junk food. Either way, you will benefit greatly from skilled surgeons using the latest techniques guided by the most up-to-date diagnostic equipment. These areas of medicine are the best ever. It's just those patent medicines we have a big problem with.

The focus of this book isn't just health. It's health with plenty of energy to do whatever it is we want to do while we're here. And *bursting with energy* doesn't come from surgery or the latest diagnostic equipment. Energy comes from applying the basic principles taught in this book.

When I'm at a convention for natural medicine (original human blueprint) doctors, I'm always happy and never disappointed when Dr. Shallenberger speaks to us. I always learn something from his insights.

I'm sure you will too!

Jonathan V. Wright, M.D.
Tahoma Clinic, Renton, Washington (www.tahoma-clinic.com)
Author, *Why Stomach Acid is Good For You, Maximize Your Vitality and Potency for Men Over 40*, and *Natural Hormone Replacement for Women Over 45* (All written with Lane Lenard, Ph.D.)

Acknowledgments

There are so many aspects that go into writing a book that have nothing at all to do with the author.

First of all, I thank almighty God for giving me the wisdom to see these truths even before there was a scientific way to verify them.

Next, I must thank all those researchers and seekers of truth who have, through their hard work, paved the way for my understanding of energy and its critical importance to health.

A special thanks also goes out to Norman Goldfind for publishing this book, and helping to get this information out to so many people who would otherwise never have heard it.

And lastly, to my editor, Roberta Waddell. I appreciate all your help with this book. I know it is much better for your input.

Introduction

I've been practicing medicine for almost thirty years, the last twenty of which have been devoted to researching and developing alternative medical strategies to increase the length and quality of my patients' lives.

Frequently, my patients ask why I decided to pursue alternative medicine. It's a good question. Especially since, when I first began to investigate this field, there was a stigma attached to it. Most doctors regarded it as quackery. The softer terms, *complementary medicine* and *alternative medicine*, had not yet been coined.

Times have certainly changed. Now there is an Office of Alternative Medicine at the National Institutes of Health. Hundreds of books have been written about alternative medicine, and even the *Journal of the American Medical Association*, a leading voice of mainstream medicine, has dedicated whole issues to the subject.

Many states have even passed legislation protecting doctors who use alternative medicine from unfair persecution by the medical boards. But the climate was totally different, and actually hostile, back in the late seventies when I first became enamored with the idea of working with natural remedies to treat and prevent disease.

SYMPTOMS IMPROVED—BUT NOT PATIENTS

After I graduated from medical school in 1973, I received training in surgery and specialized in emergency medicine. I worked in this very exciting field for the next five years and then decided I needed a change.

I chose to open a general medicine practice across the street from the hospital emergency room where I had previously worked. I naively hung up my shingle and prepared to begin a new medical career. Boy, did I have a few lessons to learn.

Within six months, I began to make the rather unsettling observation that none of my patients with chronic diseases were getting well. The ones with acute disorders—broken legs, colds, cuts, flu, and sprains—all got well, often regardless of my treatments. But my patients with chronic conditions, such as arthritis, diabetes, and heart disease, never showed any real improvement at all. Of course, with the proper medication I was able to help their symptoms. They would feel better. Their medical tests would improve. Yet the same disease process was still present.

Not only that, but many of them developed serious side effects and secondary medical conditions from the drugs I was giving them. Was I causing more problems than I was solving? Years later, statistics would become available showing that more than 100,000 people die annually as a result of *properly* administered medical therapy. But back then I was just barely beginning to appreciate the depth of this problem.

TREAT THE CAUSE, STUPID

My years in the emergency room had made me completely naive about how day-to-day medicine was being practiced on people with chronic conditions. In the emergency room, if a person was brought in with a knife protruding from his head (as actually happened once), we didn't just give him some pain medication for the symptoms and send him home. First we treated the cause of his symptoms by removing the knife and repairing the injuries. Then we sent him home.

Likewise, when a desperate patient reported he could not breathe, we quickly determined the cause, and then fixed it. We didn't just send him home with oxygen.

Emergency medicine specialists directly treat the cause of the problem, not just the symptoms. I had become so used to wondering why people have the symptoms they do, I just assumed that doctors treating chronic diseases did so as well. But I was wrong.

A few months after I launched my general medicine practice, one of my arthritis patients developed an ulcer, the result of taking a standard medication that I had prescribed. The incident alarmed me greatly. I felt I had failed this person. I decided to discuss the situation with some of the best physicians in the community at the time. I compared notes on how they treated various diseases and how I treated the same conditions, and learned I was pretty much following the conventional wisdom: ". . .We can't treat causes . . ."

I then received a life-changing piece of information from one of those doctors, a person I held in great esteem. What he told me was, "Frank, you're doing just fine. When it comes to the treatment of chronic diseases, you have to accept the fact that at this point in time we can't treat causes, because nobody knows what the causes are. The best we can do is simply make our patients feel better, and try to avoid complications with the intelligent and judicious use of medication."

Could it be, I thought, that the reason nobody knows what causes disease is because *nobody is asking the question*? This started me wondering just what kinds of things could possibly serve as causes of chronic diseases. In medical school we looked at the results of disease, the pathology. But no time was spent on the possible causes of disease.

It was around this time that I happened to pull out an old publication on vitamins that my dad had received from a drug company back in the early fifties. I started to read it and found myself devouring the information. I recall looking under the symptoms of deficiencies of different vitamins and seeing anxiety, arthritis, cancer, colitis, depression, diabetes, heart disease, hypothyroidism, rashes, and virtually every other chronic illness for which there was supposedly *no known cause.*

In the one hour of study my medical school dedicated to nutrition, we were taught that these kinds of deficiencies only occurred in serious starvation situations. They certainly did not exist among average Americans. I now began to wonder about that assumption.

THE LINUS PAULING APPROACH

In the summer of 1980, I learned about an Orthomolecular Medicine conference in San Francisco. The conference was organized by physicians who had been influenced by two-time Nobel Prize winner Linus Pauling, Ph.D. Pauling believed that diseases were caused by delicate imbalances in the body's biochemistry, and that these diseases could be prevented and often reversed simply by correcting these imbalances. He called the concept *orthomolecular* because it involved restoring the right (ortho) molecule to the body at the right time.

I anxiously went to the conference hoping to gain insight into the questions I had been pondering. I was not disappointed.

I heard about reversing, and even curing, anxiety, arthritis, gout, headaches, heart disease, hypertension, and schizophrenia merely through the scientific use of vitamins and minerals. Better yet, I learned how many of these conditions could be *prevented* using the same concepts.

I listened to medical pioneers who had been successfully using these treatments for years. I was especially happy to hear that none of these doctors were making their patients worse by creating other disorders from the side effects of pharmaceuticals. While the rest of medicine was busy pursuing the use of treatments that routinely caused death and injury from side effects, these physicians were looking for safe and effective alternatives. Although at the time I hadn't been sure where I was going in my medical career, I knew then and there I wanted to go wherever these doctors were headed.

IT'S ALL ABOUT ENERGY

Back then, except for an occasional conference like this, there was no place to learn how to proceed. There were very few books available. So I developed a set of criteria for the application of unproven, alternative techniques. First, I reasoned, they must be inherently safe. Second, they must either have a record of effectiveness, or at least be theoretically reasonable. And third, they must be inexpensive. Using these criteria as my guide, I began to take myself and my patients down an exciting and rewarding path.

Twenty-five years later, I can honestly say I made the right decision to follow this path. I have been able to help thousands of people in ways I couldn't possibly have done using only my conventional medical education.

I have learned that many natural treatments actually correct the cause of disease. I have learned that many diseases still considered incurable are, in fact, curable when the cause is recognized and treated. I have learned that virtually all the diseases so common today are easily preventable. Even aging itself is very treatable. What's the secret? In a word—*Energy*.

I have learned that a decrease in energy production is the primary cause of all diseases, allergies, fatigue, infections, obesity—and even the very process of aging. And that's what this book is all about. If you can just keep your energy production at optimal levels throughout your life, you will live longer and be healthier—and, chances are, you will never become ill.

OPTIMIZING ENERGY PRODUCTION

So, by now you are probably ready to go out to the local health food store and buy a lifetime supply of energy. Doesn't really matter what it costs.

How can you go wrong by taking a substance that is so critical to your health and well-being? The only problem is, you can't buy it. And even if you could, you couldn't swallow the pills fast enough to make a difference.

You can't buy energy—you have to *make* it. And you make it by converting oxygen to carbon dioxide. Sound complex? It's not really. In the pages to follow, you will learn exactly how your body uses this process to harness the sun's energy and make it your own.

You will learn what you can do to maximize energy production in the most efficient way possible. You will also learn about some very common bad habits that can seriously impair energy production. Knowledge is power. And you will discover firsthand the power of having maximum energy.

BIO-ENERGY TESTING

And here's some really great news. Your ability to make energy can be measured right in your doctor's office. This is done with a new testing method called Bio-Energy Testing. There are over fifteen centers right here in the United States that are offering Bio-Energy Testing. Using this technology, in about forty minutes you can determine if your lifestyle is effectively working with your genetics to produce optimal energy levels.

Not only that, if it turns out that your energy production is less than perfect, the Bio-Energy-Testing Report can often pinpoint where you are going wrong. If you are struggling with an illness, you need to maximize your energy production to get well again. And if you are fortunate enough to still be free of disease, optimizing your energy production is critical to staying that way. An entire chapter is devoted to this exciting new medical advancment.

Using this new form of energy measurement, I've been able to establish optimum values related to your energy quotient (E.Q.), your metabolism, your fat-burning ability, and other key markers that can help you hone in on optimal energy production.

HOW THIS BOOK WORKS

In Part One, I'll share these target values with you, so you will have a set of physiological references for your E.Q. if you wish to pursue the path of high energy.

With the Bio-Energy Testing method, outlined in Chapter 7, I have been able to quantify and confirm the effects of all the age-defying, energy-enhancing secrets in this book. It offers the most complete and exact measurement of health and aging I have ever encountered in all my years of practicing preventive and anti-aging medicine.

I will next discuss toxicity—what it is, how it can completely compromise your energy-producing mechanisms, and what you can do about it. I'll also explain how decreased energy production causes aging, disease, and weight gain.

In Part Two, I will sequentially unfold the clinical secrets with you. There are eight of them. They involve lifestyle changes, some very simple, some involving a bit of effort on your part, but all hugely rewarding. These secrets have the potential to raise your energy to a level you may have experienced only in your younger days, or in many cases, to a height you never imagined possible. The goal is to be *bursting with energy* for a long, long time.

THE FUTURE IS HERE, NOW

Anti-aging research has demonstrated that the human equivalent of living a fully functional life for a hundred and fifty years can be achieved in animals. Not surprisingly, the secret is energy production. In one particular study, those animals with the highest levels of energy production lived 46 percent longer than those wth the lowest levels. Even more important than living longer, the quality of their lives was much better. They were free of disease, and of course had much more energy.

The new medical specialty of anti-aging medicine is now spurring this research on and making it an increasing reality for humans. The American Academy of Anti-Aging Medicine was formed in 1993 in response to growing interest among physicians and researchers. There are now hundreds of physicians all over the world who are board-certified specialists in Anti-Aging Medicine.

Ronald Klatz, M.D., president of the organization, predicted in 1999 that a full "50 percent of all baby boomers alive and well today will celebrate their 100th birthday with physical and mental faculties intact." The question is, if you are a boomer, will you be among them? And if you are, how will you feel? To maximize your chances, maximize your energy. Please read on to see just how you can do that.

PART ONE

You Are Your Energy Level

1

Energy Production: The Real Generation Gap

HARRY, BEFORE

Five years ago, Harry was seventy-seven. He went to his doctor complaining of fatigue, insomnia, lack of stamina, stiff achy joints and muscles, weakness, and a decreased interest and enjoyment in life.

His doctor ran the usual battery of tests, and told Harry the one thing he really didn't want to hear: "You are perfectly healthy for your age." Harry knew better. He knew that "perfectly healthy" did not describe him. He left the doctor's office feeling depressed. If this was what it was like to feel perfectly healthy for his age now, what did the future bode?

Harry was a man of action, and always had been. He wanted more out of life, no matter what age he was. Drawing on an inherently resilient nature, he shoved aside the depression, discarded the doctor's verdict, and came to me for help, telling me in his first visit that he was setting out to recharge his battery.

HARRY, AFTER

Today, Harry is eighty-two and his batteries are definitely recharged. His energy production resembles that of someone thirty years younger rather than someone his age. He exercises daily and has 18-percent body fat and good musculature. His balance is good. He still backpacks up the same trails that he trekked more than half a century before. He cycles, roller-skates, and skis with ease.

He sleeps well, averaging eight hours of good sleep a night. He wakes up feeling fresh and full of vigor. His mood is exceptional. His mental-function tests reveal a fully functional brain with scores almost as good as

those of a twenty-two-year-old. He has passion for life, and is always keen
to engage and solve new problems.

He has full sexual function, and his muscles and joints are flexible and
free of the pain and stiffness that so many of his contemporaries experience. In short, Harry is living his life at an optimum level.

CAROLINE, BEFORE

Caroline was pretty messed up when she came to see me. She had just
passed her forty-sixth birthday, and for the previous five years, she had
been plagued with depression, fatigue, insomnia, menstrual disorders, and
all sorts of aches and pains. She had gained thirty pounds for no apparent reason, and couldn't lose weight even with exercise and a good diet.

She had seen several different specialists who variously diagnosed her
with chronic fatigue syndrome, depression, fibromyalgia, and hypothyroidism. More than once she had been told to remember that she was not
getting any younger, and that for her age she wasn't really all that bad.

Caroline's symptoms were different from Harry's, but the doctors were
giving her the same age-related nonsense. They prescribed antidepressants,
pain pills, and sleeping pills, but never gave her any hope for curing or
reversing her problems. In fact, they didn't even seem to know what was
causing her problems in the first place.

Like Harry, she found herself depressed by her medical treatments. What
kind of future did she have, she wondered, if she was already feeling this
bad before turning fifty?

When I first tested Caroline, her energy production was equivalent to
that of a ninety-two-year-old. "No wonder I feel like an old lady," she
lamented. "From all functional aspects, I am."

But that was then.

CAROLINE, AFTER

Today, Caroline, like Harry, has remade herself. First I confirmed her low-
energy status. Then I pinpointed the problems causing it, and designed a
program to correct them. Her many problems included a deficiency of
adrenal and thyroid hormones, along with improper breathing, poor fitness, and too much stress.

Caroline lacked the energy to fight off an ordinarily benign virus, the
Epstein-Barr virus, EBV for short. This bug is often cited as the culprit in

chronic fatigue states, which is why the condition is now generally known as chronic fatigue syndrome. Her previous physicians had focused on eradicating the virus rather than the real cause of her real problem—an energy deficit that weakened her immune system.

Caroline's thyroid function was low, which, unfortunately, had not been recognized by her doctors. They missed the diagnosis because, as is often the case, they failed to rely on the time-honored practice of taking a history and performing a physical examination along with metabolic testing. Instead, they relied exclusively on blood tests, which are often inaccurate. Caroline's test results fell in the normal range, despite the fact that her symptoms, physical findings, and metabolic tests confirmed she had hypothyroidism (low thyroid).

When the body is under stress, the adrenal glands produce special hormones that help it deal with the stress. Like most sick people I see, Carolyn was also experiencing adrenal exhaustion—illness is often the result of stress, and stress depletes the adrenal glands.

Additionally, the symptoms from the illness were causing even more stress, which was *further* draining her adrenal glands. She was not tested for adrenal exhaustion because conventional doctors are not trained in this disorder. Thus, another key to her recovery had been overlooked.

Within six weeks of instituting a program that treated all these abnormalities, however, her energy testing showed improvement. And, after another three months she began feeling energetic for the first time in many years.

Six months later, Caroline had lost thirty pounds and was back to working fulltime. Her energy production was now that of a forty-three-year-old, and she had developed an entirely fresh and enthusiastic attitude toward life.

AGE-RELATED SYMPTOMS

Before she remade herself, Caroline was a relatively young person with the energy level of a much older person. And after he remade himself, Harry was an older person with the energy production of a much younger individual. These may be dramatic cases, but many of you may be able to identify with their so-called age-related symptoms.

Harry and Caroline's symptoms are collectively known as age-related because they result solely from the aging process itself. Age-related symptoms are not caused by any disease or psychological condition. Another

way of putting it is that, in conventional medicine, you can have all of these
symptoms and be considered perfectly healthy for your age.

Common age-related symptoms include the following.

※ Anxiety and depression

※ Decreased balance

※ Decreased clarity, memory, and mental speed

※ Decreased concentration or focus

※ Decreased energy levels

※ Decreased immune function

※ Decreased sexual desire and function

※ Digestive disturbances

※ Dry, loose, wrinkled skin, and age spots

※ Hair loss

※ Increased joint and muscle pain

※ Insomnia

※ Urinary and bladder disorders

※ Vision and hearing impairment

※ Weakness, fatigue, and decreased stamina

※ Weight gain and increased body fat

For most people, the aging process begins around age thirty-five. For
some it begins earlier, for others much later. And after it starts, it may be
five or ten years before any symptoms are noticed.

Lifestyle factors, such as diet, exercise, and smoking, have a significant
influence on when symptoms show up. Long before you actually see the
first signs of aging, the process has begun, and your age-related symptoms
are on the way. It's not a case of *if*, it's simply a case of *when*.

WHAT'S YOUR E.Q.?

Caroline, Harry, and every other person with age-related symptoms, no
matter what the age, all have one thing in common—*decreased energy pro-*

duction. That decrease in energy production stems from a loss in the efficiency with which the body produces energy from oxygen.

My term, Energy Quotient (E.Q.), refers to your body's ability to produce energy from oxygen. A high E.Q. means you are doing this very efficiently. A low E.Q., on the other hand, represents a real energy crisis.

HIGH E.Q. AND LOW E.Q.

A high E.Q. means you are producing energy from oxygen very efficiently. A low E.Q. means your energy production is inefficient, and represents a real energy crisis. Just as you want your I.Q. (intelligence quotient) to be high, you also want a high E.Q.—the higher it is, the healthier you are.

If you'd like a dramatic insight into what a low E.Q. feels like, just hold your breath while reading the next few sentences. Since efficient energy production is 100 percent dependent on the presence of oxygen, you will very quickly feel the effects of a low E.Q.

Of course, decreased energy production from a decreased E.Q. is not quite as drastic as holding your breath. It is much more subtle. Sometimes my patients with a modestly decreased E.Q. feel fine. Often, they are even able to exercise as well as ever, and only in the most severe cases do they complain about being short of breath. If the oxygen levels of their blood and tissue are tested, the results are almost always normal, and yet their cells may be slowly starving for the basic energy requirements that can only be met by an optimal E.Q.

To understand how this can occur, you will first need to learn four things.

1. How the body uses oxygen to make energy.

2. What factors interfere with this process.

3. What happens when this process becomes inefficient.

4. How to improve and optimize the process.

This book will give you this vital information.

LIVE OLD—DIE YOUNG

The consideration of decreased energy production as a cause of aging and the symptoms of aging is overlooked in medical practice today. Even in geriatrics, the specialty that focuses on older people, the main emphasis is simply on treatment of symptoms. It is primarily among physicians like myself, who are interested in anti-aging concepts, that you will find any recognition and application of this energy-production concept.

Twenty-five years ago, when I first became interested in preventive medicine, nobody had much of a clue about this. I vividly remember my dad, who practiced medicine for more than half a century, telling me, "Your patients are going to die anyway. The only thing you are going to accomplish is that they are going to die in better shape." "That's precisely the point," I replied.

Of course many of us in the anti-aging field are interested in increasing the length of our lives. Life is much too precious to throw away even a day. But we should never lose sight of the fact that it is much more important to live well than to live long.

I personally hope to do both. I envision myself passing away in great shape. Free from the diseases, incapacity, and limitations that so frequently affect the older population. Science is clearly showing us this goal can only be accomplished by maintaining the energy-production efficiency we had in our youth, even as we grow very old. It is true that the younger you are when you first start making the changes, and the longer you stay with them, the more effectively they will work for you. I tell everyone not to wait until they are dragging before they decide to improve their energy production. Sure, even if you start very late in life, it will help, but the earlier you start, the more substantial your results will be.

Feeling young is a lifetime endeavor. Make it habitual, and you will live longer. More importantly, you will enjoy your life more. The purpose of this book is to help you do exactly that.

WHAT THIS BOOK CAN DO FOR YOU

If you are presently healthy, vigorous, and operating on all cylinders, you've probably got a pretty good energy quotient (E.Q.). You're bursting with energy. And the information on these pages can help you function even better and keep you at that optimum level for all the years to come.

If you are less than vigorous and energetic, suffer from ill health, or are over the age of fifty and not very active, you likely have a sub-optimal E.Q. You're bursting all right, but without energy. The information I present can help you improve your energy quotient, enhance your body's self-healing mechanisms, and slow down your rate of aging.

You won't find any of this information in another book, or in the medical library. It is based on years of working with my patients and learning the secrets that improve their energy production, health, and vigor—at all ages.

As you read through the information, you will note how the various components work together in a classic holistic sense. In other words, how you eat affects how you exercise, how you exercise affects how you sleep, how you sleep affects how you view life, and how you view life affects how you eat and exercise.

For this reason, I would like you to regard the individual secrets in this book as threads in a fabric. You are the weaver. You take the threads. You put them together and they produce a beautiful fabric. Incorporate them comfortably into your life in stages, but make sure your ultimate goal is to eventually include all of them.

It's important not to feel overwhelmed and think you need to adopt them all at once. You will be pleased to observe, as I guide you through one, then another, that your energy level is getting better and better already. And you'll be hooked.

Energy can be very addictive, you see. If you follow the guidelines, I promise you'll become an energy addict. Making you one, and making you healthier and more youthful in the process, is why I have written this book.

2

How Your Body
Makes Energy

Your body produces energy two ways, aerobically and anaerobically. Aerobic production refers to energy that comes from oxygen, while anaerobic production is energy created without oxygen. The two mechanisms are totally different, so take a moment and see how they work. Aerobic first because that's the most important process.

THE AEROBIC PROCESS

Inside the trillions of cells in your body, molecules of oxygen, hydrogen, sugar, fat, vitamins, minerals, and amino acids pass through an assembly line of enzymatic processing that generates an enormous amount of energy. About 60 percent of this energy is used to produce heat. The remaining 40 percent is used to fuel every single physiological and biochemical reaction in your body.

A fairly reliable way to determine your aerobic-energy production is to gauge how easily you become chilled, or notice if your body temperature is below normal. Yet another indicator of low aerobic-energy production is the most frequent complaint doctors hear from their patients, "I feel tired."

Poor production of aerobic energy causes a decrease in energy that results in much more than simply being tired and cold. *More than any other single factor, this is the underlying cause of aging, disease, and weight disorders.* The term that I coined, E.Q. (energy quotient), refers to the ability to produce energy aerobically.

EQ = AEROBIC ENERGY PRODUCTION EFFICIENCY

Remember when you could easily bounce up three or four flights of stairs? Now you get winded after even one or two flights. That's because your E.Q. has decreased. As you age, your E.Q. steadily falls in a very predictable manner. This decline is a solid indicator of your functional age—the age level your body is functioning at.

And here's a key point—anything that improves your E.Q. makes you functionally younger.

THE ANAEROBIC PROCESS

Anaerobic metabolism is a way for the cells to get extra energy without using oxygen. Nature designed it for emergencies, such as when trying to escape from a lion that has you in its sight for the next meal. It kicks in when a very high amount of energy is needed for a very short period of time.

Anaerobic-energy production normally occurs on a limited basis as an everyday part of cellular function, and is considered completely normal and healthy. However, when aerobic-energy production is decreased, as measured by a low E.Q., anaerobic production is increased to make up for the deficit. And this increased level of anaerobic-energy production is what accounts for many of the aches, pains, and other infirmities doctors routinely see.

A common reason for the development of a low E.Q. and the subsequent increase in anaerobic-energy production is a decreased delivery of oxygen to the cells. Another is a loss of function in the mitochondria, the energy-producing structures inside cells. Both situations routinely result from a number of sources, including the following.

☀ Deficient dietary protein

☀ Dehydration

☀ Excessive dietary carbohydrates

☀ Hormonal deficiencies

☀ Improper breathing

☀ Inadequate sleep

☀ Poor fitness

☀ Poor nutrition

☀ Sunlight deficiency

Here's why the anaerobic process is much less desirable than the aerobic process.

☀ It generates only a fraction of the energy produced by the aerobic process.

☀ It generates a high level of free radicals, highly destructive molecules that damage cells and their genetic material. Free radicals are considered a major cause of accelerated aging.

☀ It also creates high levels of lactic acid. You already know what lactic acid feels like. It is a waste product of anaerobic-energy production that causes the breathlessness, fatigue, and muscle pain that occurs with exercise. As your E.Q. decreases, you will begin to have these symptoms even with lower levels of exertion because the body is simply losing its ability to produce energy aerobically, and is forced to rely more on anaerobic production.

As the process of aerobic-energy production becomes compromised, your E.Q. slips, and you start to feel and see the effects of aging.

DECREASED E.Q. = INCREASED AGING AND DISEASE

Whether it is a brain cell sparking a thought, or a stomach cell initiating your digestion, every aspect of your physiology is 100 percent dependent on aerobic-energy production. Your liver is crucially dependent on it, as is your hair and skin, your sex organs, your strength, your vision—*everything*.

Nothing is as important to your health and your experience of life as the energy you produce from oxygen. Without aerobic-energy production you can't think, move, reproduce, resist infection, detoxify yourself, or make a structural protein or enzyme. *You can't do anything.*

And overwhelmingly, every disorder that people develop as they age is associated with an insufficient E.Q. This is why I have spent the last seventeen years researching how to both measure and improve E.Q. What I have learned through clinical experience, including feedback from my patients and research, I am now passing on to you.

Ever wonder why young people rarely develop disease despite their typical excesses, stress, lack of sleep, the worst of diets, and even smoking? How do they manage to stay out all night long and come back for more activity the next day? The answer ultimately lies in their incredible E.Q. Once you understand the factors involved in how your body uses oxygen to make energy, you will see how it is possible to maintain a youthful E.Q. even as you grow older, thereby avoiding disease and slowing down the aging process.

THE OXYGEN ODYSSEY

All energy production starts with the sun. Its radiant energy is picked up by plants and, through a process called photosynthesis, is used to convert carbon dioxide into oxygen. This oxygen is then released into the air. All living creatures inhale the oxygen and convert it back to carbon dioxide. In the process, aerobic energy is produced.

Plants keep the process of life going by continually using the sun's energy to convert the carbon dioxide that is produced back into the oxygen that is crucial to life. So, next time you feel the sun's rays, or see a tree, be sure to offer thanks because all life on earth depends on them. If it were not for the plant kingdom's recycling of carbon dioxide into oxygen, all living beings would have long ago used up all the planet's oxygen and become extinct.

Depending on where you live, the air you breath contains from 20–23 percent oxygen. If you live in a metropolitan area, or at a high altitude, there will be less oxygen in the atmosphere. If you live at sea level, or in a rural area with lots of trees and vegetation, oxygen will be more abundant. No matter where you live, however, your body adapts to the level of oxygen that is present.

Step 1—Your Lungs

The first step in the utilization of oxygen is taking in a breath. This draws oxygen into the lungs where it can be picked up by the blood.

In this process, oxygen binds to the iron in hemoglobin, a protein present in red blood cells. The oxygen is then transported by the hemoglobin to all the cells in the body. The more hemoglobin you have, the more oxygen you can take into your body.

Cigarette smoke and other forms of atmospheric pollution bind up a percentage of the hemoglobin, and interfere with its ability to take up and carry oxygen. Smoking just one cigarette, for example, significantly reduces the oxygen-carrying capability of hemoglobin for about forty-eight hours.

Lung diseases, such as asthma, bronchitis, and emphysema, decrease the blood's ability to pick up oxygen from the lungs. Additionally, improper breathing is a very common cause of decreased oxygen uptake in the lungs (more about this in Chapter 13). But, assuming you don't have a lung disease, don't smoke, don't live or work in a contaminated environment, and you breathe correctly, you will be able to saturate your hemoglobin with oxygen. This is the first step to assuring yourself an optimal E.Q.

Step 2—Your Heart

From the lungs, your oxygenated blood then travels to the heart, which works non-stop to pump blood throughout your body. A heart that pumps optimally helps you meet your energy needs in two ways. First, by sending your oxygen-saturated blood out to your body's tissues, and second, by returning it to the lungs to pick up another load of oxygen. The heart's stroke volume is the amount of blood pumped with each beat. Obviously, the heart is going to be able to deliver oxygen more efficiently when its stroke volume is optimal. In connection with this, the more you exercise, the greater your stroke volume.

The other important factor for optimal heart efficiency is the heart rate. The faster the heart is capable of beating, the more oxygen it can deliver. Both stroke volume and maximum heart rate decline with aging and with decreased fitness. Conversely, both improve with anti-aging therapy and fitness programs—another good reason to exercise.

Step 3—Your Arteries

In this delivery system, the heart is only half of the equation. Your arteries are the other half. It is the arterial system that carries the oxygen from the heart to the tissues and cells. Although your heart is a pump, unlike a centrifugal pump which has a constant output, it pumps in beats. For maximum efficiency, therefore, the arteries need to be flexible so they can expand to accommodate the sudden increase in pressure when the heart pushes out a volume of blood. Then, when the heart relaxes between beats, the arteries must contract back to their original shape in preparation for the next beat.

This flexibility of the arteries is just as important to adequate circulation as the heart itself. When arteries lose flexibility and become constricted due to stress, aging, and other factors, the result is an elevation of blood pressure. This is why blood pressure goes up in most people as they get older.

The degree to which your blood pressure becomes higher than it was when you were younger is important. It reflects how much flexibility your arteries have lost. And even though your readings may still be in the so-called acceptable range, if they are higher than they used to be, your circulation has been compromised.

Although blood-pressure readings are a good indicator, there is now a more sensitive way to measure the loss of arterial flexibility. It is called arterial-stiffness measurement. Using these measurements, decreased arterial flexibility can show up even in those who have normal blood pressure readings.

Additionally, because their stroke volume is so low, people with a poorly conditioned heart can have normal blood pressure even when they have significant arterial stiffness. In these cases, their blood pressure may not become elevated until they begin to exercise.

When deposits of plaque develop on arterial walls, a condition known as atherosclerosis develops. It results in a hardening and narrowing of the arteries that further chokes the blood supply. When this condition becomes advanced, it can set the stage for deadly heart attacks or strokes.

Step 4—2,3 DPG

Your oxygenated blood courses through many thousands of miles of arteries and arterioles (smaller arteries) until its gets to the capillaries, which are the tiniest level of all the blood vessels. The capillaries are where the real action is. It is in the capillaries that the hemoglobin will release the oxygen in order for it to be taken up by the cells. And, in this process, a special enzyme called 2,3 DPG becomes critical.

This enzyme, 2,3 DPG, forces the hemoglobin to release its tight hold on oxygen. If there is insufficient 2,3 DPG, the hemoglobin riding aboard the red blood cells would simply cruise right on past the cells and back to the heart without giving up its oxygen payload.

People who don't exercise regularly, or who have elevated insulin levels or diabetes, have decreased levels of 2,3 DPG. This makes their cells unable to obtain enough oxygen, even in the presence of the normal functioning of their lungs, heart, and arteries. Although their blood-oxygen levels may be quite normal, this can be very misleading because, even though the oxygen is present, it can't get into the cells. And when oxygen can't get to the cells, you might as well be holding your breath.

Step 5—Your Mitochondria

The delivery addresses for oxygen in your body are the mitochondria located in the cells of your body. These microscopic structures are the power plants of the cells. Inside them, oxygen, carbohydrates, and fats are processed by special enzymes. This complex process leads to the production of the aerobic energy I have been talking about. Besides producing energy, the mitochondria also produce water and carbon dioxide as by-products.

The mitochondria are very complex structures influenced by diet, genetics, and hormones. As people age, these cellular dynamos become especially vulnerable to damage. Anti-aging experts believe that the decrease in energy production caused by damaged mitochondria is responsible for all the diseases, frailty, and infirmities so typical of the aging process.

HOW YOUR MITOCHONDRIA ARE UNDERMINED

Because of the importance of optimal mitochondrial function to your health, I want to focus on what causes mitochondria to operate less efficiently, and eventually leads to their destruction.

Decreased Fitness

The most critical factor in mitchondrial function is an adequate delivery of oxygen. This means there needs to be plenty of iron and hemoglobin, good lungs, adequate breathing, good heart function, flexible arteries, and plenty of 2,3 DPG. The key to all these factors being optimally maintained is regular, efficient exercise.

When people are sedentary and unfit, and especially if they smoke, they are dramatically decreasing the efficiency of their mitochondria. No wonder it is so uncommon to hear a person who exercises regularly complaining of poor energy. No wonder it is so uncommon to hear about a person who exercises regularly coming down with a disease. (*See* Chapter 13, Secret Six, for detailed information on exercising properly.)

There is no question about it, lack of proper, regular exercise is the single most important way to decrease mitochondrial efficiency. But there are many other factors that also undermine the mitochondria. By paying attention to all these factors, you can be sure that your mitochondria will be operating just as efficiently as they did when you were young, even as you grow very old.

Hormonal Deficiency

Your body has an inner intelligence that regulates all of its functions. And no body function is more important than energy production. This is where hormones play their most important role—your body uses hormones to regulate energy production.

When the body needs more energy, certain hormones, called catabolic hormones, turn on cellular energy production just as a light switch turns on a light. If there is a deficiency in any of these hormones, the cells do not get turned on, and every one of the body's functions becomes impaired. The most important hormones for energy production are cortisol, growth hormones, insulin, progesterone, testosterone, and thyroid hormones. In Chapter 15, I will tell you how to keep these hormone levels youthful, even into old age.

Adrenal Insufficiency

After lack of exercise and hormonal deficiency, the most common reason for decreased mitochondria function is a shortage of glucose (sugar). This deficiency occurs as the result of poorly maintained blood glucose levels— a condition referred to as hypoglycemia. Hypoglycemia is a condition, not a disease, and it exists to one degree or another in just about everyone with any medical disorder. It can even be found in healthy people, where it is the single most common cause of fatigue.

Every cell in the body has the ability to create energy from either glucose or fat. Every cell, that is, except brain cells. For the most part, brain cells can only utilize glucose. Therefore low blood glucose affects the brain far more than it does the other organ systems, and is the most common cause of brain dysfunction.

Because blood glucose is so important, the body is blessed with two glands which see to it that adequate glucose levels are maintained at all times. These are called the adrenal glands. They are located just above your kidneys on either side of your mid back. The adrenal glands are quite small, but they pack a very big wallop.

If you are exercising and rapidly using up your blood-glucose levels, your adrenal glands will secrete just the right amount of the hormones cortisol and adrenalin. These hormones will see to it that the levels remain rock steady. Even in conditions of starvation, your adrenal glands will make sure that your body has an adequate supply of glucose. No matter what the circumstances, through the action of cortisol and adrenalin, your adrenal glands will be there for you, to make sure your cells are getting as much glucose as they need. That is, until they become exhausted.

Exhausted adrenal glands is the most common disorder doctors see. When I give lectures to doctors about how to make sure their patients are producing adequate levels of energy, I ask the question, "How can you tell if your patient has exhausted adrenal glands?" I then give the answer. "Because they are in your office." This is because, no matter what problem their body is dealing with, most people can get by until their adrenal glands become overtaxed. Once the adrenals become exhausted, however, blood-sugar levels can no longer be maintained, and their body quickly feels the effects. It is then that they usually decide it is time to see the doctor.

Symptoms such as ADD (attention deficit disorder), anxiety, depression, headaches, hyperactivity, insomnia, low energy, moodiness, and poor mental clarity and concentration are usually just side effects of adrenal exhaustion. Unfortunately, this is a diagnosis that is too often missed by conventional physicians.

And, all too often, many of the remedies that people use to self-medicate the early symptoms of adrenal fatigue involve alcohol, coffee, or sugar. Although these do help temporarily, persistent use of them only serves to further weaken the adrenals.

The ultimate result of adrenal exhaustion is decreased energy production. This is especially noticeable when exercising because, as long as the body is at rest, the mitochondria (in all cells except brain cells) can meet their energy needs from fat. But during exercise every cell relies heavily on glucose metabolism.

So, a hallmark of early adrenal insufficiency is normal energy at rest with a decrease in exercise tolerance. As the adrenals further weaken, however, low energy will be felt even when not exercising. Although there are many causes of fatigue, the fatigue of adrenal exhaustion can be recognized by the fact that it is much worse in the afternoon hours. This is due to the natural rhythm of adrenal functioning, which causes the glands to have a high level of activity in the morning and decreases as the day progresses.

Adrenal insufficiency results from chronic stress and excessive carbohydrate consumption. Let's take stress first.

Adrenal insufficiency from stress

Most physicians will tell you that, more than any other single factor, disease is caused by stress. This is because stress depletes the adrenal glands, and depleted adrenals add up to low energy production.

Stress comes from many sources and in many forms: mental and emotional, allergies, dehydration, drugs and pharmaceuticals, illness, inadequate rest, infections, injuries, nutrient deficiencies, pain, sunlight deficiency, or toxins. Thanks to the adrenal glands, the body is well-equipped to deal with all these stresses. As the various stressors act to put the body into a state of imbalance, the adrenals produce hormones which put it back on track. As long as the stress load isn't too severe, or doesn't last too long, the adrenals can do their jobs. Too much stress, however, eventually results in fatigued and exhausted adrenal glands.

The late Hans Selye, M.D., who pioneered the understanding of how stress contributes to disease, confirmed in experiments how prolonged stress gradually wears out the adrenals. When this happens, they are unable to produce an adequate amount of their anti-stress hormones. Since the primary function of the adrenal hormones is to maintain a healthy glucose level, the end result of chronically overworked adrenals is low blood sugar. This, in turn, results in more stress in the form of decreased energy production, further depleting the adrenals.

Adrenal insufficiency from diet

The adrenal glands, and hence your energy production, are also compromised by a diet too high in carbohydrates and too low in fat and protein. Such a diet is typical of many vegetarians, particularly a strict vegetarian diet called a vegan diet. This type of diet can inflict major harm on the adrenals. I have only seen a handful of vegans who were healthy. This small group must be blessed with the right genetics to adapt to this unusual diet. Normally, it is just not compatible with optimum energy and performance.

Carbohydrates are particularly harmful to the adrenals. By this I mean sugar (white and brown sugar, honey, corn syrup, molasses, etc.); food items made from grains, such as corn, rice, and wheat; fruits (particularly juice); tubers (beets, carrots, potatoes, yams, etc.); and to a lesser degree, beans. Carbohydrates such as these rapidly elevate your blood sugar. This is especially true when they are consumed without adequate protein and fat to decrease their blood-sugar-elevating effect.

From what I have already said about low blood sugar, you might think eating foods that raise blood sugar would be a good thing. But you'd be wrong. A rising blood sugar level causes the pancreas to secrete the hormone insulin, and insulin acts to lower the blood sugar. This stresses the adrenal glands since, in order to prevent insulin from lowering the blood sugar too much, they will now have to produce hormones to raise the blood sugar and counteract this effect of insulin. This is how, through the action of insulin, a diet too high in carbohydrates will weaken and eventually exhaust the adrenal glands.

The Wrong Fats

So far you have learned three ways in which mitochondrial energy production can be compromised: decreased fitness, hormonal deficiency, and adrenal exhaustion. Another way is by eating the wrong kinds of fats. This is because a diet high in the wrong kinds of fats decreases the function of the cell's membranes—both the outer cell membrane and the mitochondrial membrane.

First, take a look at the effect of dietary fats on the outer cell membrane. Each cell has special gateway sites on the surface of its outer membrane called receptors. These receptors are critical to all cellular activities, including energy production, and they must be working well in order for the cell to take in fat, glucose, and nutrients. They are also critical for the functioning of hormones and other messenger molecules.

Receptors are extremely complicated structures, and there is a great deal that is not yet known about how they function. One thing medical researchers do know is that they are very much affected by the types of fats people eat, particularly the type of polyunsaturated fats. The polyunsaturated fats in the diet determine the makeup and function of cell membranes. And since the receptors reside on membranes, their ability to function well is dependent on the composition of the membranes.

Up until fifty or sixty years ago, nature primarily provided only one type of polyunsaturated fat—CIS fats. These are the fats that make up healthy functioning cell membranes. The other type, known as trans fats, occur naturally in some foods, but only in extremely low amounts. The overwhelming amount of trans fats found in contemporary diets are not there naturally. They are the result of food processing.

Food processing refers to so-called foods created in a factory by man, instead of by nature. An important part of food processing involves separating the fats found in food from the rest of the nutrients in the food. An example would be taking the CIS fats out of the safflower seed to produce safflower oil. The problem with doing this is, when the fats are separated from the other protective nutrients in the plant, they become very susceptible to rancidity. So susceptible that the shelf life of the products manufactured from them is extremely short. In only a matter of days, the fats in the products would become rancid.

So when commercially processed foods began to proliferate in the early 1900s, manufacturers needed to find a method to protect the fats from rancidity. The method they discovered involved chemically treating the CIS fats with hydrogen. The first commercial example of hydrogenated fats was Crisco. Although this treatment process, known as hydrogenation, completely destroyed the nutritional benefits normally derived from these fats, it did protect the fats from rancidity. Hydrogenation offered a long shelf life, and gave the food manufacturers who used them a better bottom line.

The problem with hydrogenating fats is that, in the process, as much as 45 percent of the CIS fats are converted to trans fats. And so the delicate balance of fats that is found in nature—primarily CIS fats, with very few trans fats—becomes completely turned around. This dramatically affects the function of the cell's membranes because the shift in the fat balance found in the diet causes a similar shift in the composition of the fats in the membranes. And researchers have shown that membranes contaminated with trans fats cannot function efficiently.

Unfortunately, hydrogenated trans fats have now become a major part of the American diet. The National Academy of Sciences (NAS) advises the United States and Canadian governments on nutritional science for use in public policy and product-labeling programs. Their 2002 publication, *Dietary Reference Intakes for Energy, Carbohydrate, Fiber, Fat, Fatty Acids, Cholesterol, Protein, and Amino Acids,* contains their findings and recommendations regarding the consumption of trans fats. The NAS concluded that "trans fatty acids are not essential and provide no known benefit to human health." They further stated that there is no safe level for eating trans fats. This viewpoint has been supported by a 2006 *New England Journal of Medicine* review that states, "from a nutritional standpoint, the consumption of trans fatty acids results in considerable potential harm, but no apparent benefit."

You can identify these harmful fats by looking at the ingredient label to see if it contains the words *hydrogenated* or *partially hydrogenated*—for example, hydrogenated soy oil, or partially hydrogenated safflower oil.

Trans-fatty acids are harmful to the cells in two ways. First, they undermine the integrity of membrane receptors. Nothing gets into the cells except through the action of these receptors. And the energetic effect of hormones, which is so crucial for efficient mitochondrial function, depends completely on the cell receptors. Secondly, because of their effects on the function of the mitochondrial membranes, trans fats block the ability of the mitochondria to produce energy. Scientists refer to this effect as *uncoupling* because it uncouples the production of energy from the metabolism of oxygen.

The bottom line? A diet containing trans fats will markedly affect how cells function, resulting in a significant decrease in mitochondrial energy production.

Inefficient Fat Utilization

For the purpose of clarity, in the remainder of the book I will refer to glucose metabolism as carbohydrate metabolism. Technically, glucose is only one example of a carbohydrate. But since all carbohydrates must be broken down to glucose before they can be used for energy, I think it is easier to refer to carbohydrate instead of always referring to glucose.

All cells, with the major exception of brain cells, prefer to burn fat rather than carbohydrates (glucose) for energy. The body evolved this way because fat is more efficiently stored, was much more available in the pre-supermarket days, and produces less acid waste than carbohydrates.

People have been led to believe that dietary fat makes body fat, but this is only half the truth. In fact, both dietary carbohydrate and dietary fat make body fat.

It works like this. When you eat, only a fraction of the food is used immediately for energy—most of it is stored as fat. That's right. If you eat carbohydrates, they get stored as fat. And if you eat fat, it gets stored as fat.

Either way, your body will store the energy content of your foods as fat.

This goes back thousands of years. Humans evolved in a world where the next meal was always in question, and they may easily have gone several days or longer without eating. That's why the body evolved its system of storing dietary calories as fat. When food was available, people ate as much as they could, and then hung on until the next meal, using the stored fat for energy in the interim.

You could ask, "What does this have to do with now? Hasn't the body evolved beyond that?" And the truth is, no, it hasn't. Genetic studies on the remains of ancient man have shown that twenty-first century bodies still have the same genetic code that existed two hundred thousand years ago.

The body can all too easily store fat, but certain factors make it hard for the body to break down that stored fat and convert it to energy. The primary factor that blocks the release of stored fat for energy is carbohydrate intake. That's right. The more carbohydrates you eat, the less fat you will burn. Another major factor is hormonal deficiencies, particularly deficiencies of the growth hormones, testosterone, and the thyroid hormones. I will cover these two very important topics in great detail in the chapters to come.

The ability to break down stored fat and get it to the mitochondria to be burned by oxygen for energy production is referred to as fat utilization. Poor fat utilization leads to poor oxygen utilization, which ultimately results in decreased energy production. This is one of the most common causes of decreased mitochondrial function.

An additional problem with poor fat utilization is that it forces the mitochondria to burn more glucose in order to generate the same amount of energy. Since the body can only store a very small amount of carbohydrates, the carbohydrate reserves become exhausted within a matter of hours, and this results in a falling blood-sugar level. When this falling blood-sugar level threatens to bottom out, the adrenal glands step in to try and restore normalcy. If this scenario is repeated too often, it will ultimately stress the adrenal glands enough to cause the adrenal insufficiency described above.

Carnitine Deficiency

The early humans ate a diet very high in meat. This meant they had an abundant intake of amino acids, the components of protein. One of the most vital of these amino acids is carnitine. Researchers estimate that early man took in around 5,000–10,000 milligrams of carnitine per day. Currently, the average intake among Westerners is more like 100 milligrams.

Why? Because carnitine is found only in animal protein, and contemporary diets have shifted away from animal protein and toward carbohydrates.

In the body, carnitine is converted into an enzyme called carnitine transferase. This enzyme is responsible for transporting fats into the mitochondria for energy production. Diets low in carnitine result in low levels of carnitine transferase in the body, and a deficiency of this enzyme—common now because of carbohydrate-heavy diets—compromises fat-burning capability.

A deficiency of carnitine will result in a significant decrease in mitochondrial function. A commonly seen indicator of carnitine deficiency is the combination of fatigue, weight gain, and an elevation in the blood of certain fats called triglycerides.

Vitamin and Mineral Deficiencies

Once fat and/or glucose are introduced into the mitochondria, they enter into an assembly-line process that eventually produces energy. In what is called the Krebs cycle (also known as the citric acid cycle), hydrogen atoms are removed from the fat and glucose molecules. These hydrogen atoms are then combined with oxygen to make water and energy. In order for the Krebs cycle to function efficiently, optimum amounts of key amino acids, vitamins, and minerals are required.

The most important nutrients are the B vitamins (especially B_6, niacin, and riboflavin), certain amino acids, and the minerals chromium and magnesium. These nutrients can easily become depleted when the body is stressed or the diet is poor. The result is decreased energy production.

Coenzyme Q_{10} Deficiency

Coenzyme Q_{10}, CoQ_{10} for short, is a vitaminlike substance that is absolutely necessary for cellular energy production. As mentioned above, after the Krebs cycle removes the hydrogen atoms from fat and glucose, they are combined with oxygen to form water and energy. This step is known as cellular respiration. The first and most critical enzyme in this process is CoQ_{10}. As people age, they become deficient in CoQ_{10}. Additionally, a poor diet can cause a deficiency, and any deficiency of this vital enzyme will greatly limit mitochondrial function.

Mitochondrial Decay

Obviously, to the degree that the mitochondria become destroyed, the entire energy process suffers. Scientists refer to this process as mitochondrial decay, and it is known to occur universally as people age.

One cause of mitochondrial decay is exposure to harmful chemicals, such as pesticides. But a more frequently occurring problem comes from the long-term impact of what are known as heavy metals. The most common heavy metals in question are arsenic, cadmium, lead, and mercury. The level of these metals in the environment has dramatically increased in the past 150 years as a direct result of industrialization. They have crept into the water and food supply to such an extent that it is simply impossible to avoid them.

Elevated levels of mercury have so widely contaminated tuna and other fish that public health authorities in some areas of the country have warned against eating more than two fish a month to avoid the hazards of their mercury content. Additionally, the mercury contained in silver dental fillings, the most common dental filling material, has been shown to leak into the body and accumulate in this fashion.

Arsenic, lead, and cadmium are now routinely found in the food and water supply in this country. Well water and tap water from the faucets of older high rise buildings can be especially problematic. Even if your current water supply is clean, you may have toxic levels in your body as a result of drinking contaminated water years ago. An exposure to heavy metals will often still be present in the body many years later because they are very poorly eliminated from the body.

But, of all the factors that lead to mitochondrial decay, the most influential one is decreased energy production. Stay with me on this, because in the next chapter I'm going to do more than just explain how this can happen. I'm also going to show you that, in all likelihood, unless you have been doing something about it, your own mitochondria are traveling down the road to destruction even as you read this book.

3

Energy and Aging

WHAT IS AGING?

Before I get into what causes aging, let me first define what I mean by the word. Misunderstanding the meaning behind the word aging often leads to a lot of confusion, even among physicians. As most people use it, the word aging is synonymous with getting older. In other words, it is an inevitable consequence of celebrating birthdays. You get older, you age. Simple. Using this definition, any discussion about decreasing or reversing aging becomes ludicrous.

But in the medical sense, the word aging takes on a slightly different meaning because, in medicine, aging is defined as a decrease in the ability of the body to function efficiently. Using this definition, a person will age only to the extent that his or her body is functioning less efficiently. Let me give you an example of how this works.

Take the case of a typical twenty-year-old man. Ten years later, on his thirtieth birthday, he is ten years older. People using the usual definition of aging would say that he has aged ten years. But if he is typical of most young men, no decrease in his body's ability to function efficiently has occurred. Therefore, from a medical standpoint, he has not aged at all.

How about when he reaches forty? Will he have aged by then? Again, the functional difference between a thirty-year-old and a forty-year-old is virtually nil, so using the medical definition of aging, he still has not aged, even though he has now celebrated forty birthdays.

Using this functional definition of aging, you can begin to see that aging is not purely a matter of getting older. It is very possible, indeed quite common, to get older and yet show no signs of aging. But let's continue with this example. What about when this man reaches fifty? Surely, by then he will have some measurable decrease in his body's functional efficiency. And the answer is, of course he will. I don't know of any fifty-year-old man with a body that functions every bit as well as it did when he was twenty. So finally, by the age of fifty, you are pretty sure to find at least some evidence of aging in everyone. Aging is certainly inevitable provided a person lives long enough. There's not much to be done about that. But what is not inevitable is the rate at which people age. And that is what anti-aging medicine is all about.

As people age, they develop what are known as age-related symptoms. These are the symptoms that result as the body begins to lose it functional efficiency. In other words, age-related symptoms are not caused by a disease or a psychological condition. Another way of putting it is that you can have all of these symptoms and *be perfectly healthy for your age.*

Common age-related symptoms include vision and hearing impairment; anxiety, depression, and insomnia; weakness, fatigue, and decreased stamina; increased body fat; decreased sexual desire and function; dry, loose, wrinkled skin and age spots; and decreased memory, mental speed, and clarity. In addition to these symptoms, aging also renders everyone significantly more susceptible to Alzheimer's, dementia, cancer, cardiovascular disease, and all the other diseases that occur with greater frequency as people get older.

WHAT CAUSES AGING?

There have been dozens of theories attempting to explain what causes the decrease in function that defines the aging process. These include the free-radical theory, the Hayflick limit theory, the neuro-endocrine theory, the mitochondrial decay theory, the telomerase theory, and the wear-and-tear theory, just to mention a few. For a good descriptive synopsis of all of the various theories of aging, refer to *The New Anti-Aging Revolution* (Basic Health Publications, 2007), an excellent book on anti-aging medicine by Drs. Ronald Klatz and Robert Goldman.

Each theory has its own special attraction and logic. And each theory leads to a particular line of therapy designed to retard or reverse aging. But a very practical problem that all theories of aging have in common is that their effects can't be measured, so there is no good way to determine whether the therapies stemming from any of these theories are actually working.

If you adhere to the free-radical theory of aging, for example, you believe that aging is caused by a certain class of molecules called free radicals. Proponents of this theory believe that by decreasing the amount of these molecules, it is possible to slow down the aging process. But since it's not possible to measure the amount of free radicals in either an animal or a person, it's impossible to determine if any given line of therapy is actually decreasing free radicals. And hence, impossible to validate whether or not the theory actually holds water.

Similarly, those who believe in the telomerase theory have the same problem. They believe that aging is the result of accumulated damage in the end section of a chromosome called the telomere. Telomeres protect the genetic code from being altered during the cell's replication cycle. Therefore, damage to the telomeres will result in loss of genetic code, presumably causing aging. Unfortunately, since there is no way for you to see the doctor and have your telomeres tested, there is no way to determine whether or not the anti-aging measures you are taking are actually protecting your telomeres. Further, even if what you were doing was working, there is still no way to determine if it is slowing down the aging process.

Regrettably, the sobering truth is that each and every theory of aging is plagued with the same curse—*there is no good way to determine whether or not it actually has value in the real world.*

THE ENERGY-DEFICIT THEORY OF AGING

One of the best-studied aspects of the aging process is that the older a person is, the less capable she or he is of making energy. To use my terminology, the older you are, the lower your E.Q. becomes. According to the mitochondrial decay theory of aging, this decrease in energy production is caused by the destruction of the mitochondria. In other words, as you age and lose your mitochondria, you will not be able to produce energy as efficiently—which is to say, *aging causes low energy production.*

My research, using Bio-Energy Testing, has led me to a very radical departure from this conventional assumption. The results of my experience after testing and improving the energy production of hundreds of individuals has lead me to formulate an entirely new model of what causes aging—one which offers a unique perspective on aging and what can be done about it.

In short, my new model is this: The decrease in energy production that is observed in all aging animals and humans is not only a result of aging, it is also the cause of aging, which is to say, *low energy production causes aging.* Put another way—to the extent that an individual can maintain optimum energy production as he or she grows older, that person will not age.

Take a look at how this new idea of mine, which I call the Energy-Deficit Theory, explains all of the other theories of aging.

The Telomere Theory

According to the Energy-Deficit Theory, it's not that damaged telomeres result in aging and decreased energy production. Rather it is decreased energy production that leads to damaged telomeres and aging. How? When telomeres become damaged, as they do routinely during the cell's replication cycle, they are repaired by telomerase enzymes. These enzymes are 100-percent dependent on energy production. In the absence of adequate energy production, telomerase enzymes can't be fully effective, and the result is damage to the telomere.

The Free-Radical Theory

According to the Energy-Deficit Theory, it's not free radicals that result in aging and decreased energy production. It's decreased energy production that leads to free-radical damage and aging. How? Free radicals are natural by-products of normal energy production. But when energy production becomes less efficient, free-radical production escalates dramatically. Combine this with the fact that free radicals are reduced by certain enzyme systems called antioxidant enzymes. And, as with all enzymes, the synthesis, maintenance, and function of these antioxidant enzymes are completely dependent on energy production. Therefore, when energy production is decreased, antioxidant enzyme function is decreased, and free-radical-induced tissue destruction escalates.

The Neuro-Endocrine Theory

This theory states that aging is caused by a natural decrease in the sensitivity of hormone receptors in the brain. Proponents have evidence that this results in decreased hormone production, which in turn leads to aging and decreased energy levels. But hormone receptors are 100-percent dependent on energy production in order to function. Therefore, according to the

Energy-Deficit Theory, it is an initial decrease in energy production that causes the decreased receptor sensitivity, and that results in the decreased hormone production that is so much a part of the aging process. So it's not the decreased receptor sensitivity of the neuro-endocrine theory of aging that leads to aging and decreased energy production. Rather, it's decreased energy production that causes the decreased receptor sensitivity.

The Mitochondrial Decay Theory

This theory states that the decrease in energy production seen with aging is a result of irreversible damage to the mitochondria, called mitochondrial decay. But long before there is any actual mitochondrial decay, there is already a measurable decrease in energy production. This decrease stems from a combination of all of the factors discussed in the previous chapter. And it is precisely this early decrease in energy production that ultimately leads to mitochondrial decay and aging. I will describe how this happens in the next section.

A Unifying Theory of Aging

No matter what theory of aging you examine, it can invariably be explained as secondary to decreased energy production. This is one of the most compelling and attractive aspects of the Energy-Deficit Theory. It can explain *all* the phenomena that have led other investigators to arrive at each of the other theories of aging. This makes the Energy-Deficit Theory the *only* central unifying theory of aging.

The Energy Deficit Comes First

In a paper I recently submitted for journal publication (*see* Appendix B), I describe a condition I discovered. I call it EOMD, which is short for early onset mitochondrial dysfunction. It refers to a deterioration of mitochondrial function that leads to decreased energy production.

This condition is commonly found in young, healthy people, and becomes even more prevalent with age. Deterioration of mitochondrial function is not the same as mitochondrial decay. The latter refers to the actual destruction of the mitochondria, whereas mitochondrial deterioration means that the mitochondria are there, but are not producing energy efficiently.

To investigate just how common EOMD is, I reported on fifty young people between the ages of twenty and forty who were being tested at one of several clinics routinely using Bio-Energy Testing. Each person was free of disease and felt great. They were just having the test in order to make sure that their health program was working. The results were as follows:

☀ 54 percent (27) had normal mitochondrial function

☀ 46 percent (23) had EOMD (less than 100 percent of predicted mito-chondrial function)

☀ 36 percent (18) had less than 90 percent of predicted mitochondrial function

☀ 26 percent (13) had less than 80 percent of predicted mitochondrial function

☀ 12 percent (6) had less than 60 percent of predicted mitochondrial function, and fell within the diagnostic category of severe dysfunction

The results of the study confirmed that close to half of these young peo-ple were already showing evidence of EOMD. Approximately one quarter of them had less than 80 percent of what was expected from healthy, young people. And an amazing 12 percent of them were in the diagnostic category of severe mitochondrial dysfunction.

These test subjects were much too young to have mitochondrial decay, free-radical damage, telomere damage, or any other effects of the aging process. And they were much too healthy to have cardiovascular disease, or any other disease for that matter. Yet, an alarmingly high number of them had evidence of a measurable decrease in their mitochondrial func-tion, leading to significant decrease in energy production.

The only conclusion that can be drawn from this data is that mitochon-drial decay, free-radical damage, telomere damage, and all the other con-sequences of aging and degenerative disease are *preceded* by a decrease in mitochondrial function—EOMD. Furthermore, this decrease can often be severe, and can occur in the absence of any warning symptoms.

EOMD, therefore, refers to a deterioration of mitochondrial function in the absence of true mitochondrial decay. This distinction is important because, while mitochondrial decay is irreversible, the treatment of peo-ple with EOMD reveals that it is completely reversible.

And You Can Measure It

The Energy-Deficit Theory is not only a unifying theory of aging, but, as shown in the study mentioned above, it is also verifiable. As a doctor who actually works with real people every day, by far the most exciting thing about this theory is that it can be routinely tested and measured. Using the Bio-Energy Testing technology (*see* Chapter 7), doctors are now able to determine whether or not a person has EOMD without having to wait for either symptoms or disease to show up first.

This new model of thinking has lead to some profound and very practical implications. Instead of breaking down all the symptoms of aging into their many tiny components, I can simply ask one question: How can I increase this person's energy production to match that of a younger one?

For example, if a certain herb is shown to increase energy production in a particular individual, then I know it will decrease her or his rate of aging. Similarly, if a particular practice, such as meditation or careful limited sunbathing, can increase energy production, then it will also slow down aging.

Using this newfound capability, I have been able to discover what remedies and practices increase energy production, and which ones seem to have little effect. In this way I don't have to guess if a particular diet, therapy, or practice is going to slow down an individual's aging process. If it works to increase energy production, that's all I need to know.

The Energy-Deficit Theory in Action

Mitochondrial energy production is the single most important aspect of health, aging, and degenerative disease. But don't just take my word for it. The medical literature is loaded with proof. Take, for example, an article which appeared in 2000 entitled "Meta-analysis of the age-associated decline in maximal aerobic capacity in men: relation to training status." This research paper, dramatically demonstrates the relationship between health and mitochondrial efficiency.

In the article, using technology very similar to Bio-Energy Testing, the researchers determined the aerobic capacity in men who exercised extensively, and compared it to men who did not exercise as much. Aerobic capacity means the maximum amount of energy that can be produced by the mitocohondria. It is just another term for E.Q.

According to the authors, "Maximal aerobic capacity (a really excellent E.Q.) is an independent risk factor for cardiovascular disease, cognitive dysfunction, and all-cause mortality." This is medicalese for, "Your E.Q. will determine your likelihood of getting heart disease, dementia, and every other disease that can kill you. It will also determine this risk independent of any other factors, including cholesterol levels, diet, smoking, or anything else. This is a very powerful statement.

Then they addressed the subject of aging in particular. According to their findings, although most aspects of aging can be reversed with physical fitness training, "there continued to be a significant decline in aerobic capacity" even in health conscious, endurance-trained men as they got older. In other words, there is no better assessment of aging than optimal mitochondrial efficiency as determined by E.Q. All the other measurements of aging, such as body mass composition, bone density, cardiovascular function, or insulin resistance, can be reversed by training. Therefore, they are simply measurements of conditioning, not aging per se. On the other hand, a person's E.Q. cannot be trained away, so it represents the best measurement of health and aging.

In another article, using a different technique, the researchers examined the mitochondrial efficiency in twenty-nine men and women of different ages. Some were as young as sixteen, and some were in their nineties. They noticed a significant and consistent decline in mitochondrial efficiency with age. Across the board, the older a person, the lower their E.Q. was.

The scientific literature is loaded with studies such as these. And every single one demonstrates the integral role that decreased mitochondrial efficiency plays in the aging process. Some of them even show how certain cell functions shut down as a result of decreased mitochondrial efficiency. These functions include the ability of the body to detoxify itself, repair damaged tissues, replicate DNA, maintain water balance, and even control higher order processes, such as thinking and remembering.

THE PROOF

Two recently published studies prove that decreased mitochondrial-energy production is the primary cause of aging. In the first study, the mitochondria of certain mice were genetically altered to self-destruct much faster than normal. The researchers then compared these altered mice to mice with normal mitochondria. By now you can probably guess what happened.

The normal mice lived much longer than the ones with the rapidly deteriorating mitochondria. That was because their mitochondria were functioning much better. But even more interesting was that the altered mice not only died sooner, but they also showed all the signs of aging at a much earlier age. In other words, they were aging prematurely. They developed all the signs of aging, such as anemia, degenerated joints, hair loss, heart enlargement, muscle loss, osteoporosis, and reduced fertility, and they developed them at a much younger age. The authors concluded that the results of the study very clearly demonstrated how decreased mitochondrial function causes aging.

In a different study, scientists measured the resting mitochondrial function in a group of mice. They then observed the mice over the course of their lifespan and compared how long each mouse lived to what its mitochondrial function was. The mice with the highest mitochondrial efficiency lived *36 percent longer* than the mice with the lowest. Experiments such as these provide proof that aging and longevity are simply a matter of energy production. If you want to live a long time, and be fully functional and healthy, you better make sure that your mitochondria are functioning optimally.

Everyone agrees that unless you die young, aging itself is inevitable. At some point in time, if you live long enough, you will become feeble and then die. However, the dramatic rate and extent of aging that is commonly seen today is not inevitable. There is no reason at all that, barring serious genetic disorders, each and every person can't live to be at least 110 years old and be fully functional. The secret? As you grow older, be sure that you do whatever it takes to maintain youthful mitochondrial function. More than anything else, the rate and extent of aging depends on it.

This is also true of all the diseases that occur as people get older, diseases such as Alzheimer's, cancer, diabetes, heart disease, and Parkinson's. The literature is very clear. The single best way to prevent the diseases of aging is to maximize mitochondrial function.

BUT IS IT REALLY POSSIBLE?

In June of 2000 I was invited to speak at The First International Learning Conference on Anti-Aging Medicine in Monte Carlo, Monaco. My subject was how to set up an anti-aging clinic.

There was a fairly large contingent of physicians from China, where the government is interested in establishing a network of such clinics. During the question-and-answer session following my talk, one of these physicians asked me if I really thought it was possible to halt, and even reverse, the aging process.

My response was, it is not only possible, but, in fact, I was already doing it in my clinic in Nevada. I then explained my theory that the single best determinant of aging is the measurement of how efficiently an individual is able to produce energy.

I went on to describe how, with proper testing, it is now possible to measure anyone's energy-production efficiency (their E.Q.) quickly, easily, and with great precision. "With this method," I told them, "I have found that many of my sixty and seventy-year-old patients [who follow the anti-aging guidelines discussed in this book] are now producing energy as efficiently as a forty-year-old. I believe that these people have literally slowed down aging to a snail's pace."

Someone once said that as soon as you are born you start dying. This isn't quite true because the dying part doesn't really start until somewhere around the age of forty, but the point is well taken nonetheless. After age forty, unless something is done about it, the body's cells enter into deterioration mode, and with time, the rate of decline accelerates. This is called aging.

Have you ever asked yourself how and when you want to die? If you haven't, I think you should. The reason is this—if you want to live a long and fully functional life, there are many things you must do (or stop doing, as the case may be) *before* you experience the symptoms of aging. And the time to take action is right now. The younger the better.

Someday I will die, but until then I want to live as healthy and vibrant a life as possible. I don't want arthritis, cancer, dementia, diabetes, or heart disease. I especially don't want the feebleness and frailty that is often considered an inevitable part of hitting the eighties. And throughout my professional life, it is this strong desire that has compelled me to discover as much as I can about the aging process. How to slow it down, and how to prevent the diseases of aging. I now know that, to a very large extent—barring an accident or an act of violence—it is possible to determine not only how and when we will die, but more importantly how long and how well we will live.

THE GOLDEN YEARS?

A patient once told me that the golden years were when you needed more gold. More gold to pay for doctors, medications, and nursing homes. This concept of what it's like to get old is so universal that when I first begin to discuss the idea of living longer, many people say they are just not interested.

"I'll deal with that later," they often say. "Why bother myself with that while I am still feeling well? I want to focus on the positive. And besides, no one wants to live forever."

True, no one wants to live forever. But just about everyone would like to live their golden years free of the diseases and frailties that so commonly characterize this period. Free to feel young, be employed, go fishing with great grandchildren, hike up a mountain, have sex, maybe even go back to school—or just free to really enjoy another beautiful day.

It seems that Mother Nature really plays a dirty trick on everyone. She weakens and deteriorates people just when they have gained the wisdom and experience to really appreciate the beauty that life has to offer. Just as they realize that being alive and feeling strong is a blessing, they are rudely interrupted by a damaged heart and the need for someone to drive them to the cardiologist.

ME, 100 YEARS OLD!?

They say you could live to be more than a hundred years old. And they're right. According to the World Health Organization, "There have been more gains in life expectancy in the last fifty years than in the previous five thousand years."

The U.S. Census Bureau has gone on record as saying that, "By the year 2025 there will be two sixty-five-year-olds for every teenager in America." So the odds are looking better and better that you will live to be quite old. The question then becomes, what do you want it to be like, and what can you do about it.

Recent advances in medical research have shown that much of the mental and physical decline traditionally perceived as the inevitable consequence of aging can be delayed, prevented, and often even reversed. Many doctors are realizing that aging is a treatable condition, just like any other physical disorder.

The diseases associated with aging are preventable. So, too, is the functional decline in mental and physical ability. The disabilities you have been so used to seeing in older people do not have to be a part of your life.

Perhaps the best news is that achieving these benefits is becoming easier. Moreover, you don't have to be rich to make the golden years really golden.

4

Energy
and Disease

If you want a change, you have to change.

Einstein once said that the definition of insanity is repeating the same thing over and over again and expecting a different result. If that's the case, then our current system of medicine is clearly insane.

If the way you live has brought you to the diagnosis of a disease, then according to Dr. Einstein, it would be insane to treat the disease without changing the way you live and expect a different result. That is unless you want to keep the disease. If you want to keep the disease, it makes good sense to keep on living the same way.

But I can't completely blame the medical system for this insanity. Much of the blame must go to human nature. Human nature makes people lazy and resistant to change. Human nature makes people want that bypass surgery, and gets them to somehow deny that unless they change the way they live, they'll be having another one in five to six years.

Human nature says, "Doc, just please cure me. Cut the problem out. Give me that magic pill, and don't tell me I have to change anything. I want to be healthy and still maintain the same lifestyle that made me sick in the first place".

It is now known that all the diseases of aging are completely preventable. How? By maintaining optimal energy production as you get older, which involves being smart, and changing the way you live. In this chapter, I address specific issues related to the prevention and treatment of our most common age-related diseases—cancer, cardiovascular disorders, diabetes, and osteoporosis.

CARDIOVASCULAR DISORDERS (ATHEROSCLEROSIS, STROKES, AND HEART DISEASE)

Vascular disease, also known as arteriosclerosis, develops when blood vessels become hard, stiff, and inflexible. If this occurs in the major arteries leading to the heart, brain, and legs, the consequences can be serious and life-threatening.

The most common type of this disease is atherosclerosis, a term adopted from the Greek words *athero* (paste) and *sclerosis* (hardness). The Greeks had it right. In this condition, plaque deposits form on the inner lining of the arteries. They are made from fat, mostly cholesterol, and then become hardened by the deposition of calcium. The result is a hardening and narrowing of the arteries and the reduction of vital blood flow. This reduction in circulation deprives cells throughout the body of oxygen and essential nutrients. When this process becomes advanced in arteries leading to the heart, you can develop chest pain (angina) and heart attacks—the number one killer. When the process involves arteries leading to the brain, or small arteries within the brain, you can develop a stroke or senility.

Atherosclerosis is also a major contributor to premature aging because the decrease in circulation means that less oxygen and nutrients are reaching the cells for energy production.

Scientific evidence indicates that atherosclerosis is completely preventable. *When I say completely, I mean 100 percent.*

With what we currently know, this condition and all the diseases associated with it, can be completely eradicated. But to understand how to eliminate the problem, you must first have an understanding of what causes it.

WHAT CAUSES ATHEROSCLEROSIS?

When asked, most people would say that the villain is simply too much cholesterol in the blood from too much cholesterol in the diet. This answer contains but a small shred of the truth. *Cholesterol is only one of many different factors, and is, in fact, a relatively minor one at that.* It is not the *Great Satan of Heart Disease,* as we have been led to believe.

The beginnings of atherosclerosis occur with damage to the inner lining of the artery. The primary factor involved in this initiating injury is decreased energy production, and many of the causes for this decrease are well-known. Happily, all of them are treatable.

Exaggerated Stress Response

Hardening of the arteries seems to be accompanied by a hardening of attitude. As people get older, they tend to react more to stress than when they were younger. This results from an accumulation of attitudes, such as inflexibility, clinging to grief, guilt, old hurts, a lost sense of purpose, regrets, decreased appreciation of beauty, and fear of death and disease. Over the years, this kind of stress wears out the adrenal glands, and decreases blood flow to the cells, causing a measurable decrease in energy production. Chronic stress also causes adrenalin-induced free-radical damage, increased cholesterol, and high blood pressure, all of which damage arteries.

There are many cures for dealing with stress. Meditation. Exercise. Rest. Spending quality time with grandkids or friends. Pursuing a hobby that unleashes unexpressed creativity within you. Good companionship. A pet. No matter how old you are, or what misfortunes have befallen you, the key is finding things in life that bring you joy and nourish the heart and mind. This is what dissolves stress.

Over the years, Dean Ornish, M.D., has published amazing studies clearly demonstrating that coronary artery disease can be reversed by stress-management techniques, such as meditation and yoga, along with proper diet and exercise.

Hormonal Deficiencies

The most significant hormone deficiencies leading to atherosclerosis involve DHEA, estrogen, growth hormone, testosterone, and thyroid. These hormones are critical for optimal maintenance of energy production. As you get older, these hormones will become deficient. It's not a question of *if* they become deficient, it's only a question of *when*. And as their levels start to fall, you will be at greater risk for developing atherosclerosis. Natural hormone replacement is one of the most effective ways to keep your arteries soft and pliable (*see* Chapter 15, Secret Eight).

Mineral Deficiencies

A proper diet minimizes the risk of mineral deficiency. However, due to commercial farming methods, the use of synthetic fertilizers, and the processing of food, meals often end up short of the key minerals that contribute to healthy arteries. The most common deficiencies I find among my patients are chromium, magnesium, and zinc.

Having these minerals in your body in adequate amounts is critical for optimal energy production. Chromium is especially important for fat metabolism. And zinc and magnesium are key to mitochondrial function. The medical literature is replete with studies connecting deficiencies of both chromium and magnesium to atherosclerosis.

In one study, every single person with coronary artery disease was found to have low chromium levels, whereas only 20 percent of those without the disease had low levels. Animal studies have also demonstrated a 50-percent reduction in atherosclerotic plaques in animals given supplementary chromium.

According to an article appearing in the prestigious cardiovascular journal, *Circulation*, magnesium deficiency is associated with an increased risk of coronary artery disease, myocardial infarctions, fatal arrhythmias, and sudden cardiac death.

Using a new technology, electron beam coronary tomography, researchers have been able to document that coronary artery disease is directly correlated with increased levels of calcium in the coronary arteries. Magnesium supplementation has been shown to decrease the calcium content of these arteries, making them much less likely to develop atherosclerosis.

Regular supplementation that includes these minerals is critical for maintaining your health, even if you think you are eating a perfect diet.

Chronic Heavy Metal Poisoning

In the previous chapter, I discussed the toxic effects of chronic heavy metal exposure on the ability to produce energy. These toxic metals in the air, water, and foods can build up in the body over decades, and when they do, they poison the mitochondria. Arsenic, cadmium, and lead, in particular, contribute to arterial damage. The most common source of these metals is drinking water. This is very good reason to make it a habit to drink only filtered water.

Once inside your body, the heavy metals get deposited in the tissues, particularly the arteries, where they accumulate. They cannot be readily excreted and they will not be detectable using standard blood and urine tests that are used to discover acute heavy metal poisoning. Their presence in the body can only be discovered by what is called provocative testing. This is a technique offered by many practitioners of alternative medicine, which involves the administration of chelating substances that bind to heavy metals stuck in the arteries and other tissues, and promotes their excretion through the urine.

By obtaining a urine specimen before and after the chelating substance is administered, it is possible to ascertain the full extent of the heavy metal poisoning. The pre-provocative urine specimen will show few, or no, heavy metals, while the post-provocative specimen will be loaded with them. This demonstrates two principles connected with heavy metals.

1. Simply examining the blood or urine for heavy metals without using a provocative chelator is basically useless for documenting their presence.

2. Without the continuous use of chelation, the heavy metals won't be removed.

Inadequate Sleep

Lack of adequate sleep is a documented cause of diabetes, hypertension, and obesity, all of which are contributors to atherosclerosis. Why? As you will see in Chapter 9 (Secret Two), sleep deprivation is one sure way to markedly decrease your body's energy-producing capability.

Poor Cardiovascular Conditioning

This means insufficient exercise—specifically, not enough of the right amount and right kind of exercise. (*See* Chapter 13, Secret Six.)

One thing that Bio-Energy Testing routinely discovers is how poor the typical over-fifty heart is at providing adequate oxygen to the cells and tissues. One group of cells, the intimal cells that line the arteries, requires a very high level of oxygen to properly function. Because these cells cannot optimally function without adequate oxygen levels, and this makes them especially vulnerable to the various processes that cause atherosclerosis.

Regular exercise to the rescue here. Of all of the measures you can do to improve your energy production regular exercise is by far the most effective. It can prevent, and even reverse, poor cardiovascular functioning by providing increased levels of oxygen to the intimal cells, and thereby reduce atherosclerosis.

Obesity and Insulin Resistance

I lump these two together because they are almost always found together. In Chapter 5 you will learn that both conditions occur as a direct result of decreased energy production. You will also learn how to diagnose them, and how to treat them by increasing your body's ability to produce energy.

Elevated Homocysteine Level

Homocysteine is a naturally occurring amino acid in the body. Under normal circumstances, it is rapidly cleared by the liver with the help of vitamins B_6, B_{12}, and folic acid, and food substances known as methyl donors. However, any deficiencies of these vitamins, and/or sub-optimal liver function can result in an elevated homocysteine level. And that spells trouble.

The excess homocysteine triggers harmful reactions that initiate damage in the arterial walls. Studies confirm that about 10 percent of all deaths from atherosclerosis occur as a result of an elevated homocysteine level.

People with a close relative who developed heart disease before the age of sixty often have elevated homocysteine levels. This buildup can be counteracted by maintaining a healthy liver, and supplementing with the key vitamins listed above.

Excessive homocysteine also has damaging effects beyond the arteries. According to a study in the *Annals of the New York Academy of Sciences*, it can also cause chromosomal damage, which is a major sign of aging. Other studies have shown that people with even a moderate elevation of homocysteine have as much as a 50-percent increased risk of dying from all causes of illness than those with the lowest levels. The lab reports the statistical range of homocysteine to be between 5 and 15 umol/L, but optimal levels are below 7 umol/L.

Excessive homocysteine levels are commonly associated with decreased energy production. This is because homocysteine levels become elevated as a result of a deficiency of the metabolic process called methylation. As such, an elevated homocysteine level often means that adequate methylation is not taking place.

Methylation is a process that occurs in every cell in the body. It involves the transfer of methyl groups (three hydrogen atoms attached to a carbon atom) from one molecule to another. This methylation transfer is critical for many important functions, including detoxification, mental and emotional functioning, and energy production.

In terms of energy production, methylation is absolutely critical. This is because it is through the methylation process that all of the ADP that is made in the body is created.

ADP is adenosine *di*-phosphate. The di- means it has two high-energy phosphate bonds. As you will learn in Chapter 7, all of the usable aerobic energy produced in the mitochondria is harnessed in a molecule called ATP (adenosine triphosphate). ATP is created when the mitochondria add a third high-energy phosphate bond to ADP. Therefore, in order for the mitochondria to produce energy, they must have a good supply of ADP. An adequate supply of ADP is so critical that, without ADP, all mitochondrial energy production would immediately stop and you would instantly die.

The process of methylation is also where another important energy molecule called creatine is made. Having enough creatine around is essential for providing a steady supply of energy to your cells.

Your cells cannot store ATP for use later on. They can only use it as it is being produced. But what if your needs for energy at any given moment exceed your mitochondrias' ability to supply it fast enough? This is where having enough creatine around becomes so important.

The molecule creatine offers a way for the cells to store the high-energy phosphate bond found in ATP for later use. It works like this. Once ATP is formed (from ADP), it can then cause its high-energy phosphate bond to react with creatine. In this process, the phosphate gets transferred to creatine to form creatine phosphate. Since the ATP loses its phosphate bond in the process, it is converted back to ADP, thereby supplying the mitochondria with more ADP to create energy with.

Unlike ATP, creatine phosphate can be stored for later use. So when the cells need a sudden amount of ATP, as is so often the case, they don't have to wait for the mitocholndria to produce it. They can get it instantly from their supplies of creatine phosphate. They simply reverse the above process, and transfer the high-energy phosphate from the stored creatine phosphate back to an available ADP molecule to create an instant supply of ATP.

Thus, creatine plays an essential role in the maintenance of an adequate supply of ATP. When there is not enough creatine to go around, the availability of ATP becomes very compromised, and cellular function suffers.

Now you can see why it is so important to make sure that your homocysteine levels are optimal. Because optimal levels are a good indication that your body is methylating well, and producing enough ADP and creatine. These molecules play critical roles in the production of optimal energy.

Lipoprotein (a)

Elevated blood lipoprotein (a) has received less attention than homocysteine, and much much less than cholesterol, but it is nevertheless a significant risk factor for heart disease. The best way to make sure your lipoprotein (a) levels are low is to pick your parents well. That's because lipoprotein (a) levels are genetically determined.

This substance is an extremely sticky molecule. As it circulates in the blood, it has a marked tendency—greater than any other lipid—to adhere to sites of arterial-wall damage and contribute to plaque buildup, arterial blockades, and atherosclerosis. You know that the higher your cholesterol levels are, the greater your risk for atherosclerosis. But what you probably don't know is that 46 percent of cholesterol is made up of lipoprotein (a). And it is the lipoprotein (a) part of the cholesterol and LDL cholesterol molecule that is responsible for its damaging effects.

For the same reason that lipoprotein (a) causes heart disease, it is also associated with developing a condition called intermittent claudication. People with intermittent claudication notice muscle cramps in their legs after walking only 100 yards. Lipoprotein (a) also interferes with the clotting mechanisms of blood, causing it to clot more easily. This creates an additional risk factor for heart attacks and strokes.

The acceptable statistical range for lipo (a) is up to 80 mg/dL (some labs report as high as 130 mg/dL). But the optimal level is much lower. Most authorities state that the healthiest levels of lipoprotein (a) are below 20 mg/dL.

Linus Pauling, one of the greatest scientific geniuses of the twentieth century, argued almost thirty years ago that an elevated lipoprotein (a) level was the leading risk factor for heart disease.

You haven't heard more about this substance for a simple reason. Big Pharma (aka the drug companies) hasn't yet been able to patent a drug to decrease it. When this happens, as it no doubt will, you can expect a high-decibel campaign about a completely new discovery—a sad commentary on the way medicine is practiced in this country. Instead of being driven by physicians and their patients, who care the most, medicine today is driven by pharmaceutical corporations whose overriding interest is the bottom line.

The good news is, you don't have to wait for the drug industry, there are already some excellent solutions. They're not patentable, but they work. Years ago, Pauling discovered that lipoprotein (a) damages the arteries and causes atherosclerosis by adhering to a part of the inner lining of the arteries called the lysyl residues. But lysyl residues are also present on a common amino acid called l-lysine. Pauling was able to show that taking l-lysine as a supplement diverts lipoprotein (a) from adhering to the lysyl residues in the arteries towards adhering to the lysyl residues contained in supplemental l-lysine. Taking l-lysine won't lower your lipoprotein (a) levels, but it will protect your arteries from it.

Another amino acid called n-acetyl cysteine can also help. One study showed that n-acetyl cysteine, taken as a supplement, was able to lower lipoprotein levels as much as 70 percent. This is particularly effective when the n-acetyl cysteine is combined with vitamin C.

In men, one of the causes of increased lipoprotein (a) is a deficiency of the male hormone testosterone. If you are a man with elevated levels of lipoprotein (a), be sure to have your testosterone levels checked. If they are low, replacing your sagging levels with natural testosterone will help to lower lipoprotein (a). I will discuss this in much greater detail in Chapter 15.

With the additional support of B vitamins, proper exercise, and a low-carbohydrate diet, this dangerous sticky stuff can be kept in its place.

Coenzyme Q_{10} Deficiency

CoQ_{10} is a vitaminlike substance. It is a fundamental enzyme in the cellular conversion of oxygen to energy. Therefore, any decrease of it threatens your energy production and promotes the possibility of many related problems. Depletion is associated with aging, poor diet, the use of cholesterol-lowering drugs, diabetes, and heart disease.

Adequate CoQ_{10} is necessary for the integrity of all tissues—and even more so for those tissues with a high metabolic need for energy, such as the brain, heart, and liver. Studies show that people with heart disease are deficient in CoQ_{10}, leading to decreased heart function. And, according to Texas cardiologist Peter Langsjoen, M.D, who has been using CoQ_{10} in his practice for more than twenty years, a CoQ_{10} deficiency can also lead to high blood pressure.

CoQ_{10}, which often becomes deficient as you age, is made in the liver from the less complex forms found in foods, such as CoQ_6 and CoQ_8. Yet another reason why your liver is the most important organ in your body. The statistical range for levels of CoQ_{10} is between .75 mg/ml and 1.5 mg/ml, but most research indicates that levels above 2.0 mg/ml are required for optimal health. I strongly recommend supplementing with CoQ_{10} to remedy any deficiency, and I particularly recommend it for people who are middle-aged or older.

Anyone taking a cholesterol-lowering statin drug should definitely be on a CoQ_{10} supplement because statins block the synthesis of CoQ_{10} and often result in dangerously low levels. Blood levels should be checked to be sure that the dose is adequate. The failure to do so means substituting one relatively minor risk factor (cholesterol) for a much more significant one (a CoQ_{10} deficiency).

Elevated Iron

The iron story is fascinating. Women have a much lower incidence of heart disease than men and also live an average of 10–15 percent longer. And this difference exists in every culture studied, regardless of diet, exercise, or stress. There is one exception, however—men who regularly donate blood. These men basically share the same desirable statistics as women.

Why is this so? It might be because of iron. Inside the body, iron is a two-edged sword. On the one hand, it is critically important for the production of energy. Iron chemically binds to oxygen in hemoglobin molecules in the blood and carries the oxygen for delivery to the cells. But it is also iron, in excess, that instigates damaging free-radical activity.

Because of their cyclic blood loss, menstruating women have less iron. But many men, unless they regularly donate blood, have a tendency to develop higher iron levels. So do post-menopausal women who do not donate blood. Excessive iron consumption from supplements, or iron cookware, can also be a contributing factor.

Excessive iron levels can be discovered by examining the blood ferritin level. Ferritin is an iron-binding protein that stores iron in the liver. A blood test revealing too high a level of this substance indicates an excess of iron in the body.

I routinely check the ferritin level of my patients and find that 10–15 percent of men and 3–5 percent of post-menopausal women have elevated levels. I make sure these patients are careful about their dietary intake of iron. I also recommend that they donate blood regularly, as this is the surest way to maintain optimal iron levels. In addition, natural substances, such as algae, colostrum, garlic, and inositol hexaphosphate (IP_6), are able to lower iron levels.

In most labs, the reported range for serum ferritin levels is usually between 40–180 ng/ml. But in my opinion, and that of many experts in this field, any value over 70 ng/ml can indicate an excessive amount of iron in the body.

Antioxidant Deficiencies

I have already discussed free radicals, the highly reactive molecular fragments formed in the course of everyday energy production in the cells. In excess, they cause considerable damage to cells and tissues, and are major factors in disease processes and accelerated aging. Free radicals, for example, are always involved in the initial arterial damage that leads to atherosclerotic plaques.

The body has evolved an elaborate defense system of enzymes and other substances called antioxidants to prevent a harmful excess of free radicals. This system is stimulated by aerobic exercise and weakened by stress and infection. It is also undermined by exposure to pesticides, petrochemicals, and other chemicals.

Certain nutrients are required to keep the antioxidant system running strong. Among these are vitamins, minerals, and amino acids. Fortunately, these substances are widely available in health food and drug stores. Chief among them are vitamins C and E, CoQ_{10}, alpha-lipoic acid, the amino acid cysteine, and the minerals copper, manganese, selenium, and zinc. These supplements can help your body's fight against free radicals, and can also help prevent the development of atherosclerosis.

Elevated Blood Triglycerides

Triglycerides are fats produced in the liver from carbohydrates. The more carbohydrates you eat, the more triglycerides you will make. An elevated

ative of eating a diet too high in carbohydrates, and increases r cardiovascular disease.

lence of triglycerides on atherosclerosis seems in large part related to HDL, the so-called *good* cholesterol. High triglycerides cause a decrease in HDL. Harvard researcher Michael Gaziano, M.D., pointed out the significance of this relationship in a 1997 article in the cardiology journal *Circulation*. He found that individuals with the highest ratio of triglycerides to HDL were sixteen times more likely to have a heart attack than those with the lowest ratio. Ideally, triglyceride levels should be below 120 mg/dl. An ideal HDL/triglyceride ratio is 1/2. A ratio of less than 1/3 should be treated.

Improving this ratio can be readily achieved through weight loss, exercise, a low-carbohydrate diet, and supplementation with fish oils and niacin.

Hypertension

The relationship between hypertension and atherosclerosis is well known. Simply put, elevated pressure in the arteries is a significant cause of atherosclerosis.

More than 50 million Americans have this condition, also called high blood pressure. Your blood pressure should ideally be at or below 120/80. If it is higher than this, the standard treatment is anti-hypertensive medication. However, strange as it may seem, many of the medications used to treat high blood pressure actually promote atherosclerosis—this is particularly true of beta-blocker and diuretic medications.

In most cases, hypertension responds well to a combination of treatments focusing on weight loss, exercise, a low-carbohydrate diet, and supplementation with CoQ_{10}, fish oil, and magnesium. Breath meditation (*see* Chapter 14, Secret 7) is also beneficial because it helps relieve stress, a major contributor to hypertension.

Stress is often related to time urgency, the feeling there just isn't enough time to accomplish what needs to be done. It will always be more attractive for the time-urgent individual to take a blood-pressure pill in three seconds than to alter the diet, meditate, exercise, and take supplements. But for those who really want to live longer and better, the correct choice is clear.

For anyone with severe hypertension who has been on medication for many years, it may be difficult to eliminate the drugs. But the alternative approach often allows a reduction in the medication.

The Great Cholesterol (Mis)Conception

Cholesterol is obviously involved in atherosclerosis, but not to the degree you have been led to believe. The whole issue of cholesterol has been overblown, oversold, and totally distorted as a public menace. It has become a fixation of the medical establishment and has spawned a huge industry. You have low-cholesterol foods. No-cholesterol foods. Cholesterol blood tests. And most troubling of all, there is the increasing promotion of a very dangerous class of drugs called statins to lower cholesterol levels. The ads are everywhere: on TV and radio, and in newspapers and magazines.

These drugs are even being promoted to healthy people as a smart prevention strategy. A strategy for what? For making big pharmaceutical companies richer, that's my opinion.

There are many good reasons why fixating on cholesterol, and worse, trying to lower cholesterol with drugs, is a dangerous and medically unsound way to prevent heart disease. Here are five important ones.

Reason 1

❊ Cholesterol is only one of many factors leading to heart disease. If all the risk factors aren't individually identified and treated, simply lowering cholesterol will not appreciably reduce your overall risk.

❊ Studies *repeatedly* show that these medications demonstrate no beneficial effect at all for 70 percent of those who use them. The other 30 percent show a modest benefit at best.

❊ Many of the studies examining the effect of lowering cholesterol on the overall incidence of heart disease have been quite disappointing. One of the first and largest of such studies is the Helsinki and Oslo Heart Study. This study showed there was a 34-percent decrease in coronary heart disease from the cholesterol-lowering drug. However, despite this, there was no reduction at all in deaths in the cholesterol group. Worse than that. The non-illness death rate (suicides and accidents) was more than twice as high in the drug group. Sure they had less heart disease. That made their cardiologists happy. But they were pretty much dead anyway. Why? Because maintaining adequate cholesterol levels is critical to maintaining adequate brain function. Similar results were also seen in the Lipid Research Clinics Coronary Primary Prevention Trial, and many other studies.

Reason 2

※ It is not actually cholesterol per se that damages the arteries. *It is oxidized cholesterol.* Cholesterol becomes oxidized when the body's antioxidant defenses become depleted. This occurs as a result of excess stress, inadequate fitness, and deficient intake of antioxidant nutrients. Ironically enough, cholesterol drugs actually suppress a major component in your protective antioxidant defenses, CoQ_{10}.

※ Following the steps in this book can help prevent cholesterol from becoming oxidized, thereby preventing your high cholesterol levels from harming your arteries, no matter how elevated they are.

Reason 3

※ The most common cholesterol medications are called statins. Statins are dangerous. They have a long list of serious side effects, some of which persist even after the drugs are withdrawn. Statin drugs inhibit the enzyme system that produces coenzyme Q_{10}, a vital compound that has indispensably essential roles in the body. CoQ_{10} serves as raw material in the cellular production of energy and is a powerful antioxidant.

※ CoQ_{10} acts as a bodyguard for LDL cholesterol, accompanying the LDL in the bloodstream and protecting it from free-radical oxidation. Recent research has found that the most susceptible LDL-LDL_3—is equipped with CoQ_{10}.

※ Research has proven that statin drugs deplete the CoQ_{10} your body produces. The long-term effects of this depletion are potentially disastrous. This is what has motivated the International CoQ_{10} Association, a group of researchers and clinicians who study the uses of CoQ_{10}, to voice their concerns to the U.S. Food and Drug Administration. In 2001, these medical professionals urged that the FDA warn anyone taking statin drugs about the CoQ_{10} depletion that goes along with the drug.

※ Studies have shown that heart failure is associated with a CoQ_{10} deficiency. Heart cells require a huge amount of energy, and are therefore the primary cellular consumers of CoQ_{10} in the body. It is probable that the resurgence of heart failure in the United States is because of the effects of statin medications.

※ CoQ_{10} experts say that people taking these drugs do not develop symptoms of possible CoQ_{10} deficiency immediately. It takes about a year or two, they say, before people may start to complain of malaise and muscular aches and pains. It is interesting to note that recent medical reports have emerged about side effects of statins, and particularly the potential for muscle damage. And, remember, the heart is a muscle. In the summer of 2001, one major statin drug, Baychol, was pulled off the market by the FDA. Nobody has yet connected the dots specifically, but this could be related to CoQ_{10} deficiency. Muscles need energy to work, and without enough CoQ_{10}, energy production becomes severly hampered.

※ Not just muscles, but all cells need CoQ_{10}, and any deficiency can have widespread medical implications. For more information on the CoQ_{10}/statin connection, and for a medical update on this very important substance, you may want to get a copy of *User's Guide to CoenzymeQ10* by Martin Zucker, available in most health food stores.

※ Common complications of statins also include paralysis and rheumatic joint disease. A report in the British medical journal *The Lancet* pointed out there is no overall death-rate decrease from the use of cholesterol-lowering drugs. That's because any reduction in cardiac deaths is offset by an increase in non-cardiac deaths.

※ In fact, the sobering truth is that lowering cholesterol with drugs can actually increase the death rate. Take for example a World Health Organization study that looked at the death rates of people with high cholesterol. This study compared people taking a cholesterol drug called clofibrate to people who did not take any drugs at all, and just lived with their high cholesterol. Both groups were followed over an average period of 9.6 years. The results were startling to say the least. There were 25 percent more deaths from *all causes* in the clofibrate-treated group than in the high-cholesterol control group. No particular disease accounted for the overall excess: the clofibrate group had more deaths from cancer, heart attacks, strokes, and other major diseases. The authors of the study offered two possible explanations for the increase in death rates: 1. A long-term toxic effect of clofibrate, and 2. The unhealthy consequences of reducing cholesterol.

Reason 4

※ Common causes of high cholesterol include antioxidant deficiency, insulin resistance, low DHEA, low fiber diets, low thyroid, low sex hormones, nutritional deficiencies, and stress. If you have elevated cholesterol, you may have any or all of these problems. Instead of introducing potentially harmful drugs into the system, physicians would do better to correct the problems that cause high cholesterol in the first place. And drugs obviously don't do this, they just squelch the body's production of cholesterol, while the real causes are not addressed. In the end, the only ones really benefiting from cholesterol-lowering drugs are the manufacturers of the drugs.

Reason 5

※ The discussion on cholesterol requires a final touch to put it in full perspective. Cholesterol is in your body for a reason. It is *needed*. Less than 20 percent of the cholesterol in your body comes from your diet. Most of it is made in the liver. Cholesterol is much too important a molecule to be trusted to dietary intake alone. All your steroid hormones are made from cholesterol. All your cell membranes are made from cholesterol. And your brain and nervous system are almost entirely made of cholesterol.

※ A low cholesterol level is associated with immune deficiency and with an increased risk of death from all causes, including cancer.

To sum up, artificially lowering cholesterol is risky business. The medical profession should get off its current emphasis on cholesterol drugs and go on to more productive things.

SO WHAT REALLY CAUSES HEART ATTACKS?

I've explained the factors that cause the constriction, hardening, and narrowing of the arteries. A significant amount of blockage in the coronary arteries supplying the heart sets up the conditions for a myocardial infarction—a heart attack. But there are other factors that are just as responsible (maybe even more so) for heart attacks as blocked arteries.

Increased Clotting Tendency

Many people with coronary artery disease have a tendency to form clots at alarmingly high rates. Excessive levels of lipoprotein (a) is often one of the main reasons, but there are also other causes. This increased tendency causes extensive clots at plaque sites.

It all starts when a plaque erodes, exposing its contents to the bloodstream. The clotting elements in the blood then adhere to it. When this happens, the plaque/clot combination is referred to as a vulnerable plaque. Vulnerable plaques are dangerous. The clot part of the plaque may break off, be swept away by the blood, and cause a sudden and complete blockage of a coronary artery. The result is sudden death without any warning symptoms.

This clotting risk can be neatly reduced by taking the QuickStart and Super Fat nutritional formulas I developed (*see* Chapter 12, Secret Five). This combination contains herbs, oils, and nutrients that effectively keep the blood thin. Often, this is the only remedy my at-risk patients have to take to correct this problem.

Infected Plaques

One rather surprising cause of heart attacks involves the immune system. Researchers have discovered that common bacteria can grow on arterial plaques and infect them. As a result, the plaques may break off and cause a sudden heart attack in the same way that vulnerable plaques do.

The discovery was made when researchers found that people with coronary artery disease, who were regularly treated with antibiotics for other conditions, were less likely to have heart attacks. Apparently, those who develop these infected plaques are unable to normally mount an effective immune response to prevent the infections. The immune-enhancing nutrients found in QuickStart, along with natural homone replacement and stress reduction, can help your immune system prevent, and even eradicate these infections.

Coronary Artery Vasospasm

The coronary arteries are no different from any other arteries. They are surrounded by smooth muscles, which help to regulate the blood flow through them. When the smooth muscles constrict, they squeeze down the size of the artery and effectively decrease the blood flow. Likewise, when they relax, the blood flow is increased. Vasospasm refers to a condition in which these smooth muscles constrict and stay constricted, just as a muscle cramp does. This causes a severe decrease in the blood flow to the heart muscle. If the vasospasm lasts longer than a few seconds, it may cause chest pain and sudden cardiac arrest. Up to 70 percent of all heart-attack deaths are preceded by a coronary artery vasospasm.

Among its many important contributions to the body, the mineral magnesium helps prevent vasospasm by keeping the smooth muscles around the arteries nice and relaxed. Most coronary-artery vasospasms are caused by a deficiency of magnesium that can be caused by diuretics, a poor diet, or an excessive intake of coffee, tea, or soft drinks. Magnesium supplementation (QuickStart is high in magnesium) can significantly reduce the risk of vasospasm.

Poor Fat Utilization

An overlooked—and extremely important—factor in the cause of heart attacks is the poor ability of those with coronary artery disease to optimally metabolize fat for energy. *The heart, like all the other muscles in the body, prefers to burn fat as its primary energy source.* Anyone who has impaired fat metabolism is at a significantly increased risk for the development of a heart attack simply because the heart tissues are less metabolically active. To a large extent, this explains why people who are overweight, or have high levels of fat in their blood, are so much more likely to have a heart attack.

THE FACTS ON BYPASS AND ANGIOPLASTY

One of my major pet peeves is the escalating rise of various surgical plaque-removal procedures to treat coronary artery disease, such as bypass surgery and angioplasty. This is particularly bothersome because these procedures entail a significant risk of death and neurological impairment, combined with a high degree of failure within five years. Furthermore, they do *nothing* to address the above-mentioned causes of heart disease. There are much safer, more effective alternatives to these procedures that are readily available.

Clinical studies show no significant difference in survival rates between those who opt for angioplasty or bypass surgery and those who choose to treat their disease medically. Several years ago, the *New England Journal of Medicine* showcased a study demonstrating the ineffectiveness of either method to extend life following a heart attack.

WHAT'S ANGIOPLASTY—WHAT'S A BYPASS?

Coronary balloon angioplasty is an invasive method of opening blocked arteries that might impede flow to the heart and possibly result in heart attack or death. The technique involves inserting a tiny balloon into the affected blood vessel and inflating it. This compresses some of the blocking plaque against the arterial wall, and thus improves blood flow. Almost 1 million angioplasties were performed in the United States in 1998.

In bypass surgery, the surgeon reroutes blood around clogged coronary arteries to improve the supply of blood and oxygen to the heart. This is accomplished by taking a blood vessel from another part of the body and grafting it above and below the blocked part of the affected coronary artery. More than half-a-million bypass surgeries are performed in the United States each year.

In the study, researchers at the University of Toronto compared the death rate for 400 Canadians with heart disease to a matched group of Americans. At the end of one year following a heart attack, the death rate was the same in both countries. However, the difference between how these people were treated was illustrative.

※ Three times as many Americans had angiographies

※ Three times as many Americans underwent angioplasty

※ Almost five times as many Americans underwent bypass surgery

The Americans had three to five times as many dangerous procedures, and yet the death rate was the same. This and similar studies do not suggest there is no place at all for these procedures in the medical care of people with coronary artery disease. But the results do strongly indicate that many angioplasties and bypasses performed in the United States are ineffective and unnecessary.

The main guiding diagnostic procedure used to determine whether or not a bypass or angioplasty should be performed is an angiography. This is an invasive procedure that entails risk, albeit fairly low, of both stroke and death. It involves placing a catheter into the coronary arteries, and injecting a dye that can be seen on an x-ray. Angiographies are supposed to able to determine if the artery has a substantial blockage or not, but there are substantial problems with angiographies.

Most studies show there is very little agreement among cardiologists on exactly how to interpret the angiograms. For example, researchers at the St. Bartholomew's and the London Chest Hospitals in Great Britain randomly picked 209 angiograms that were performed in their hospitals. They then had two different cardiologists look at the angiogram results and interpret the amount of significant coronary artery disease present in each case. The results? These cardiologists disagreed in 40 percent of the cases. It gets worse. There was a 30-percent disagreement between the two specialists on whether or not a given patient should go on to have an invasive procedure or should just be managed with medication. So, depending on which cardiologist looks at the angiogram, a patient has between a 30–40 percent chance of receiving an unnecessary procedure. Other studies, also published in leading journals, have concluded that angiogram interpretation is subject to error in as many as 70 percent of the cases.

Adding up all of these studies, you can't help but reach the rather shocking conclusion that when a physician tells his or her patient that an angiogram indicates the need for bypass surgery or angioplasty, there is perhaps a 70-percent chance the interpretation is wrong. Moreover, if the interpretation is correct, the odds are only 10 percent that the bypass procedure or angioplasty will actually extend life.

How can this be? It seems so natural to conclude that if you remove the blockages, you eliminate the problem. But, as with many things in medicine, what seems rather obvious at first glance only turns out to be a small part of the whole picture.

The reason angioplasty and bypass surgery are of such limited value is because these procedures don't treat the causes, they only treat the effect.

The causes, meantime, are still at work, and the disease process is still advancing. *The most effective approach to the treatment and prevention of coronary artery disease can occur only when all causal factors are considered.* The best therapeutic approach combines the timely and judicious application of drugs and homeopathic remedies, along with attention to all the other points I have been making.

THE VALUE OF CHELATION THERAPY

Chelation therapy is the safest and most effective form of treatment for most cases of coronary artery disease. This method involves a series of intravenous infusions of minerals, vitamins, and a special amino acid called EDTA (ethylene diamine tetracetic acid).

EDTA is an amino acid similar to those found in the proteins you eat. It has a strong attraction for toxic metals, such as arsenic, cadmium, lead, and nickel, which it binds up and escorts out of the body. It also has the ability to bind up and remove calcium deposits that are hardening into arterial plaques.

Chelation improves the function of individual cells and their enzyme systems, particularly the endothelial cells that line the arteries. And it also infuses the body with beneficial minerals, such as potassium and magnesium, which are typically deficient in people with heart conditions.

Arterial walls become softer and develop greater elasticity. This increases circulation, meaning more oxygen and nutrients get to the heart and all the other cells throughout the body. And with a huge amount of toxic material being removed, the grand effect is to significantly defuse the many risk factors that lead to heart attacks and strokes.

I offer chelation therapy to my patients in the context of a broad-based healthcare approach, including the many steps outlined in this book. Along with other treatments, such as blood thinners, blood-pressure medication, and diuretics, chelation is successful in over 90 percent of all cases of coronary heart disease. Often, blood pressure is reduced or normalized, and the need for medication can be reduced or even eliminated.

An added bonus is that it improves circulation *throughout* the body, not just to the heart. You can bet that if there is atherosclerosis in the coronary arteries, it is in all the other arteries as well. In fact, I recommend that everyone receive a course of chelation therapy when they hit their sixties, even if they are healthy and free of heart disease. My thinking is that there are very few people who will reach that age without having gunked up their arteries to some extent.

Chelation therapy is effective, safe, and completely free of any significant side effects. Moreover, it is inexpensive. For those who would like to learn more about chelation therapy, not only in coronary artery disease but in other diseases as well, there are several excellent books on the subject that can be found online or in the health section of any major bookstore. To find a doctor trained in chelation therapy, contact The American College for the Advancement of Medicine at 949-309-3520 or visit the organization's website at www.acam.org.

Now for the less encouraging news—unfortunately, the method is ignored by a majority of cardiologists. In its place are scare tactics, which seem to work pretty well. I can't tell you how many times a patient of mine had been previously told by a well-meaning cardiologist that an emergency procedure is needed to "save your life."

The reality is, studies have shown that over 90 percent of all cases of coronary artery occlusion respond well to a combination of chelation therapy and medication—the only known emergency indication for surgical intervention is uncontrolled angina.

I know a number of cardiologists who are absolutely convinced that chelation therapy is not nearly as effective as angioplasty or bypass surgery. And when they see my patients, who tell them how much chelation has helped them, these doctors dismiss the improvement as a placebo effect. However, I have never met a single cardiologist who has called the method ineffective after giving it a decent chance. On the contrary, the few cardiologists I know who have been open to chelation and have given it a try, have never gone back to the knee-jerk mentality of surgery for each and every case of advanced arterial disease.

CANCER

Strictly speaking, cancer is not a disease of aging. It can strike at any age, but the incidence of the disease does rise sharply with age, which makes it reasonable to wonder what it is about the aging process that so greatly contributes to this problem.

The starting—and startling—point is this: If you are over fifty, it is very likely you already have cancer in your body. In fact, it's almost 100 percent likely. Autopsy studies of people who died in accidents, or from causes other than cancer, have confirmed that nearly every person older than fifty already has at least one cancerous tumor in the body. I am not talking about a few cancerous cells, I mean actual cancers. And, according to these studies, many were found to have more than one cancer.

If this is true, why is it that only 25–30 percent of the population dies from cancer? And why is it that many individuals live well into their eighties and nineties without ever developing any problems from the cancers that must be present in their bodies?

The answer lies in the cancer concept of *promotional factors.*

Cancer Promotion

Cancer experts say that, on average, most of us have several cells a day that mutate into a cancerous cell. The experts refer to this situation as *initiation,* and it is a normal occurrence at any age.

They also say that the immune system is equipped to quickly detect and destroy these cancerous cells before they can multiply and enlarge into a colony of cells large enough to form a tumor. Every now and then, however, a cancer cell develops the ability to elude detection and a tumor is born. It is important for everyone to realize that, in these early stages of tumor development, the tumor is far too small to be identified by any sort of medical detection.

Often, this growth is snuffed out as it becomes visible on the radar screen of the immune system. But it also may just remain there in a state of limbo—contained, but not eliminated by the body's defenses. It is this dormant stage of cancer that virtually everyone harbors, no matter what the age.

These cancers are known as *latent* cancers. Because they are so small, latent cancers can not be discovered except on an autopsy examination. You won't be aware of them. They produce no symptoms and they can't be detected by scans or x-rays. We only know they exist because of autopsy studies which use microscopic examination to find them. As far as you or your doctor know, there is no cancer present at all. And as long as your immune system is operating effectively and there are minimal promotional factors present, you will live a long, healthy life—free of any clinical cancer.

The term *promotional factors* refers to various influences and imbalances that favor the development of latent cancers into larger, clinically apparent cancers—the kind that can kill you. The precise ways these promotional factors influence cancer development are not clearly understood. But the primary central promotional factor was first proposed by Otto Warburg more than eighty years ago.

Dr. Warburg, the only physician to win the Nobel prize for medicine twice, is considered the most influential physician of the twentieth century. Dr. Warburg was able to prove that cancer cells develop primarily as a result of decreased energy production. More recent research has validated Dr. Warburg's conclusions by proving that increasing the energy production in cancer cells causes them to: a) decrease their growth rate; b) decrease their tendency to spread; and c) revert to normal cellular metabolism. In addition, increasing a cancer cell's energy production also causes it to be less malignant.

In the aging process, the immune system steadily loses efficiency. This decline, along with the decline in energy production, permits the growth of latent cancers that would otherwise be mired in the pre-clinical stage into full blown clinical cancer.

Let me share an example:

Ernest, sixty-three, came to my clinic with a problem of uncontrolled blood sugar. He had been diagnosed with diabetes several years before. It turned out the diabetes was secondary to a very rare condition created by cancer of the pancreas (the pancreas is the organ that produces insulin, the hormone that controls blood sugar). Looking back on his medical history, it became apparent that he had had the cancer for at least eight years before its presence finally became apparent.

The case is typical of newly diagnosed cancers. By that I mean the cancer is actually present and working in the body many years before any clinical indications appear. Many times physicians see patients who, only a few weeks before, were feeling fine, but suddenly have health complaints and symptoms of disease. As they investigate, the doctors discover that their bodies are literally riddled with cancer. Often, such patients have had annual physicals and blood tests that show nothing abnormal.

Experiences such as this indicate that, without symptoms, medicine is not yet sophisticated enough to recognize cancer in the latent pre-clinical stages. Once the diagnostic tools to do so have been developed, however, practitioners will be in a more advantageous position to initiate therapy before the cancer reaches a symptomatic and more destructive stage.

The Promise of an Early Detection Method

Medical science is pursuing such technology. Researchers are striving to develop reliable methods to determine the presence of cancer markers, the changes of naturally occurring substances in the blood that represent pre-cancerous development. I have already seen some promising tests and methods that give an optimistic prospect for the future of cancer detection.

One beneficiary of such budding technology has been my friend Dr. G, a pioneer in the field of alternative and anti-aging medicine. He looks about fifty, has the energy and brain clarity of a thirty-year-old, but is, in fact, seventy-two. Dr. G has been applying a variety of cancer-marker blood tests on himself for years.

Two years ago, one of these tests turned up some suspicious numbers. At first he thought the change was due to transient factors, but when the change persisted over the following twelve months, he became convinced it was indicating that a latent cancer was beginning to evolve into a clinical stage. The result didn't surprise him. His life for the past several years had been highly stressed. He had moved, set up a new clinic, started a new business venture, and typical of many in the medical profession, had too many irons in the fire.

Motivated by the results of the testing, he immediately set out to clean up his act. His efforts paid off. Within six months, the blood test results began to reverse, and one year later he tested completely normal.

Today, Dr. G is convinced he cured himself of cancer that would have become clinically detectable and potentially untreatable in three to five years. Of course such an assumption cannot be proven, but I believe he is correct.

The case illustrates two important points.

1. It is highly likely that you and I already have several if not many latent cancers. And that, under the influence of promotional factors that decrease energy production, such as stress, poor nutrition, smoking, and toxicity, these otherwise harmless cancers will evolve into a clinically detectable and potentially life threatening stage.

2. As the field of cancer-biomarker assessment further develops, we will *have the capability to detect when latent cancers are getting out of control, and treat them in their pre-clinical stage long before they reach the point of*

clinical detection. I strongly believe the coming years will bring major breakthroughs in combining blood-cancer markers with computer analysis to identify when a latent cancer is being promoted to a malignant stage.

Until that day when cancer-biomarker assessments become refined and widely available to doctors, it behooves everyone to recognize that the body harbors latent cancers and to act accordingly. This means keeping latent cancers in permanent confinement by making sure that your energy production does not decrease as you get older. Otherwise, like giving a convicted criminal the keys to the jailhouse, low energy production gives these cancers the power to break out. Following the recommendations in this book can help to keep your latent cancers in check.

OSTEOPOROSIS

Osteoporosis is a disease in which bones become fragile and more likely to break. If not prevented, or if left untreated, the condition can progress until a bone breaks, typically in the hip, spine, or wrist. The fact that women are affected four times more than men should tell you that hormones play a big role in this disease. Americans have been brainwashed into thinking that calcium deficiency is the cause of osteoporosis. This has now been proven untrue.

There are many factors in the onset of osteoporosis, but dietary calcium deficiency is not one of them. That's why taking calcium does nothing to prevent the disease. The latest study that proves this point looked at 36,282 normal healthy women between the ages of fifty to seventy-nine. These women were randomly assigned to take either 1,000 milligrams of calcium with 400 international units of vitamin D a day or a placebo. They were followed for seven years.

This extremely well done and statistically significant study found *absolutely no benefit* from calcium and vitamin-D supplements in preventing broken bones. What's more, the study showed why—only a very insignificant amount of all that calcium was actually going to the bones. The bone densities of those on the supplements showed no improvement at all in the spine. The only improvement at all was in the hip area, and it was an insignificant 1 percent.

Osteoporosis is caused by excessive calcium loss, not by an insufficient intake of calcium. That's a very important distinction to make, so I will repeat it. The problem is excessive loss, not deficient intake.

Excessive calcium loss can be quickly measured by looking for a substance called n-telopeptide in urine. This is a much more useful way to assess bone health than bone-density testing. It's inexpensive, only requires a urine specimen, and changes from therapy can be seen in less than two months. A distinct limitation of bone-density testing is that the effects of therapy can't be seen for anywhere from one to two years. This is because, even when the correct therapy is being used, the changes in bone-density measurements are so small that it takes a long time to see them. One to two years is a long time to wait to find out if a treatment is working.

N-telopeptide is a molecule that appears in the urine as a result of bone loss. The more bone loss that is occurring, the more n-telopeptide that shows up in the urine. Successful anti-osteoporosis measures will demonstrate a decrease in urinary n-telopeptide levels in only six to eight weeks. This makes it a very good way to immediately assess the effectiveness of your program.

Published studies clearly show that osteoporosis can be both prevented and treated by diet, exercise, adequate exposure to sunlight, and hormone replacement—all issues that are discussed in the book. Following these recommendations is all you need to keep your bones strong and youthful.

IS IT SAFE TO TAKE CALCIUM SUPPLEMENTS?

Calcium is the most abundant mineral in your body. Ninety-eight percent of it is used to build and maintain strong bones. Another 1 percent builds and maintains your teeth. The remaining 1 percent is spread throughout the body and serves essential chemical roles in muscle contraction, blood clotting, and the transmission of nerve impulses. Normal bone health does not just rely on calcium. Vitamins C and K also play a critical role, as do the minerals boron, magnesium, zinc, phosphorus, silicon, and strontium. True calcium deficiency is essentially non-existent in this country. It doesn't even turn up in studies of inner-city children, which have repeatedly shown that dietary intake of calcium is deficient. The reason is that calcium is the only mineral with its own regulation system. When the level of dietary calcium falls, the body compensates for this through the action of vitamin D, which increases calcium absorption from the intestines, and decreases calcium loss from the kidneys. This system works so well that a normal calcium balance will be maintained even with low calcium intake.

The author of a definitive clinical review on calcium metabolism says it best. "Many official bodies give advice on desirable intakes of calcium but no clear evidence of a calcium-deficiency disease in otherwise normal people has ever been given. In Western countries the usual calcium intake is of the order of 800–1000 mg/day; in many developing countries, figures of 300–500 mg/day are found. There is no evidence that people with such a low intake have any problems with bones or teeth. It seems likely that normal people can adapt to have a normal calcium balance on calcium intakes as low as 150–200 mg/day. This adaptation is sufficient even in pregnancy and lactation."

I believe that the *indiscriminate* supplementation of calcium to strengthen bones is not only useless, but also dangerous. You read that correctly. The food and supplement industries have achieved a major sales coup by convincing women they will develop osteoporosis unless they take calcium supplements, when nothing could actually be further from the truth.

There is not a single well-controlled prospective study showing that calcium supplementation actually prevents osteoporosis. (A prospective study means it followed the same group of people over many years—statistical studies that are not prospective are often subject to error.)

Preventing osteoporosis with calcium supplements is a nice theory, and it seems to make sense, but it just doesn't pan out. Instead of helping, supplementation can cause problems by putting an excess of calcium into the wrong parts of the body.

Can Calcium Supplements Cause Heart Disease?

What does the body do with all the excess calcium it doesn't need? It's certainly not reaching the bones. So where does it go? One common repository is the arteries. And yes, there's a connection here to arterial obstruction, calcified blood vessels, decreased circulation, and plaque.

Electron beam tomography represents a state-of-the-art diagnostic technique for coronary artery disease. Studies using this new technology demonstrate that the chances of dying of a heart attack go up in direct proportion to the calcium content of the coronary arteries. This fact raises serious concern for the cardiovascular health of people who consume large quantities of calcium supplements. Much of that calcium is just precipitating out on the arteries.

Can Calcium Supplements Cause Cancer?

What happens to someone taking supplementary calcium in spite of the fact that she or he does not have a deficiency? The first thing that happens is that vitamin-D production is suppressed by the excessive calcium intake, which leads to a deficiency of this vitamin. Since vitamin D is critically involved in proper immune-system function, all this extra calcium results in an immune deficiency which has been shown to lead to autoimmune diseases, cancer, and inflammatory bowel disease. The full magnitude of this problem remains unknown, but a glimpse into the many possibilities is provided by a paper published in 1998.

The paper, published in *Cancer Research* by the Department of Medicine at Harvard Medical School, found that the immune deficiency caused by elevated calcium intake resulted in an increased incidence of advanced prostate cancer. The authors state, "Our findings provide indirect evidence for a protective influence of high 1,25(OH)2D [vitamin D] levels on prostate cancer and support increased fruit consumption and avoidance of high calcium intake to reduce the risk of advanced prostate cancer."

Other studies show the same relationship with breast and colon cancer, and I'm sure that, because vitamin D is so important for proper immune function, in the future we will see the same problem with other cancers.

Can Calcium Supplements Cause Deficiencies?

Another problem with calcium supplementation relates to the absorption of other important nutrients. Specifically, calcium blocks the intestinal absorption sites for magnesium and zinc. By loading up on calcium, you create a deficiency of these other minerals. Many studies have confirmed that magnesium and zinc deficiencies are widespread.

What Else?

All this is bad enough, but it's not the end of the story. In the body's attempt to rid itself of excessive calcium intake, it channels the extra calcium to the kidneys for urinary excretion. And this, according to medical research, promotes kidney stones. You'll also find calcium deposits in joints and tendons, where they contribute to arthritis and tendinitis.

These facts certainly discourage me from recommending calcium supplements to my patients. With what we know about how the body deals
with calcium, it seems like wishful thinking to expect that supplementation will somehow magically restore bones without creating any of these
undesirable effects. Nor do I include calcium in QuickStart, for all the reasons mentioned.

DEPRESSION

Depression often affects older people. Why? The problems of aging, lost
vigor, and lost loved ones certainly provide ample reason to be depressed.
But these are not the major reasons. Hormone deficiencies of estrogen,
growth hormone, progesterone, testosterone, and thyroid, are even more
significant causes.

As an example, take the case of George, sixty-four-years-old. He was
reluctantly brought in to see me by his wife of thirty-six years. In front of
him, she told me, "If you can't do something about him, I am going to
lose my mind."

George had been a man of great passion and energy, but over the previous three years, he had become grumpy and complaining. Six months
prior to that, he had retired, and now he had no motivation and no interest in life.

"At least he was bearable when he was working," his wife said, "but now
that he's home all day, he drives me crazy with his complaints and
demands." George had tried counseling, to no avail. He had no idea why
he was so negative. It was completely uncharacteristic of him. Three different antidepressant medications had been tried. Each one was stopped
because of side effects, and the fact they didn't work for him.

Ordinarily, George enjoyed sex but admitted that, "If a naked super
model walked in this room right now, I wouldn't even look at her! I have
absolutely no desire for sex." During that first visit, George began to cry,
and I saw in front of me a man who had given up, who felt utterly help-
less and hopeless.

Testing revealed an abnormally low level of testosterone, combined with
an elevated level of estrogen, both common in men over sixty. Bio-Energy
Testing revealed a thyroid deficiency as well, even though his blood thyroid tests had previously been found normal.

I prescribed natural thyroid and testosterone replacement, feeling these would help elevate his depression and gusto. After three months, however, his condition had not improved, even though his testosterone level tested normal.

Growth-hormone replacement was an extremely expensive therapy at this time and for that reason I wanted to try other things first, and did not initially test him. But now I did, and not surprisingly, his growth-hormone level was quite low. I then added growth hormone to his regimen.

After one month into this expanded program, George started to perk up. When I reevaluated him in three months, his wife told me he was "almost back to his usual ornery self." Ornery or not, George was thrilled.

No counseling. No drugs. Not even exercise in his case (he was extremely resistant to that suggestion). It was just a matter of giving his body the hormones he so badly needed.

As an aside, George admitted to me that he had contemplated killing himself because he loved his wife too much to put her thought the agony of living with him. He never revealed his intention to me, or anyone, because he planned to stage the suicide as an accident so his wife would collect his life insurance.

George's case illustrates not only the powerful effect that hormones have on mood, but also the importance of prescribing *all* deficient hormones in order to optimize the therapeutic effectiveness. Since that time I have learned that testosterone replacement will often not work in the presence of a growth-hormone deficiency. Unfortunately, many physicians are unaware of the astounding impact that hormones can have on the function of the brain, and especially on mood.

DIABETES

"The latest statistics from the Centers for Disease Control indicate that nearly 16 million Americans—6 percent of the population—have diabetes, the highest level ever recorded.

Moreover, the disease is developing at the staggering rate of 798,000 new cases a year. That's equivalent to the population of Washington D.C., and about six times higher than the incidence in the early 1950s.

In my opinion, this development is a medical disgrace, a prime example of a distorted medical system that focuses almost entirely on treatment of symptoms while basically ignoring prevention. Type 2 diabetes, a disease of contemporary living, is 100-percent preventable.

A recent survey revealed that only 8 percent of Americans regard diabetes as serious. Yet diabetes is deadly serious. It is the major cause of amputations, blindness, and kidney failure in adults, and is a leading factor in disorders of the nervous system. People with diabetes are also two to four times more likely to develop strokes and heart disease.

Diabetes is caused by high levels of blood glucose (sugar) resulting from flawed insulin secretion, insulin resistance, or both. Insulin is the hormone produced by the pancreas that controls blood-sugar levels—it causes blood sugar to move into the cells for use in energy production. In diabetes, insulin function is seriously compromised.

Type 2 diabetes is the most common form of the disease and develops slowly, usually among people over forty-five who are overweight. However, health officials have started to see a disturbing increase in type 2 diabetes among children. This is a development that parallels the soaring rise of juvenile obesity. Type 2 diabetes used to be known as adult-onset diabetes, but because kids are now getting it, this term has been dropped.

The guidelines in this book will prevent type 2 diabetes, because the primary cause of the disturbance in insulin function is decreased energy production. One important must-do for anyone with diabetes is exercise. It conditions the heart and blood vessels, lowers body fat, increases muscle weight, and increases cellular uptake of insulin and nutrients.

A 1998 study published in the *Journal of the American Medical Association* (*JAMA*) suggests that even mild exercise, such as non-vigorous walking can "significantly" improve insulin sensitivity and reduce the risk of developing diabetes-related conditions.

My Recommendations to You

☀ Once you have read this book, start making the recommendations a part of your everyday life. Don't drive yourself nuts. Just start off easy, and then work into a mad frenzy later.

☀ In addition to all the important things you do for yourself to maintain optimum health, it's a good idea to visit a prevention-oriented, nutritionally-aware doctor for a regular checkup. Don't wait until you have symptoms. A prevention specialist can help identify diseases earlier, making treatment more effective, and he/she can put you on a program that further reduces your risk of developing symptoms and illness. I have screwed up my plumbing and automobile several times by trying to fix problems myself. I learned the hard way that hiring someone who knows what they are doing is essential to getting a good result. Doctoring yourself is no different. Find a good preventive physician to work with.

* Everyone over the age of fifty (that includes me) should have an annual checkup. It's the best way to keep track of your health status and monitor your progress as you strive to optimize your health. Medicine is a rapidly changing field. Every year, better diagnostic and therapeutic methods are being discovered, and it may be that your program can be improved or enhanced as a result of these developments. The annual checkup is a way to review and possibly update your program. It will allow you to find out if your preventive program is really working to make you stronger, healthier, and functionally younger. As you grow older your needs will change, and so must your program.

* Nothing is as valuable a part of an annual checkup as Bio-Energy Testing. There are more and more doctors now using this test. You can find them at www.bioenergytesting.com. If your doctor does not offer this test, please have her or him go to that website to find out how to get it. Your doctor can see a very technical explanation of the test and the science behind it by listening to one of my lectures, which is available at no charge over the Internet. The lecture can be accessed by going to www.vrp.com/webinar/archive/.

* Assume you have latent cancers and act accordingly. Promise to take better care of yourself and your immune system. Do this especially if you are going through a particularly stressful time.

* Think of your fortieth birthday as a good point in life to see a preventive doctor for baseline studies. In fact, give yourself a birthday present in the form of a baseline evaluation. This evaluation should include Bio-Energy Testing and the other important tests mentioned throughout the book. The results of these studies on your health status at forty can be used as a basis of comparison in later years as you age and embark on an anti-aging program.

5

Energy and Weight

According to government statistics, more than 60 percent of American adults are overweight. One-quarter of American adults are more than just overweight—they are obese. This puts them at increased risk for every chronic disease there is, including diabetes, heart disease, high blood pressure, strokes, and cancer. And, very sad to say, today's children are following suit. As I mentioned earlier, a weight problem among youngsters is now at an epidemic level and increasing. By all accounts, Americans appear to be the most obese people in the world, and are growing more so every year.

Obesity is not just an appearance problem, it is a huge health problem. Obesity is by far the major single risk factor for developing serious diseases. Medical experts say it is an aggravating, or independent, agent for more than thirty medical conditions.

There are many reasons for obesity. These include bad eating habits, improper exercise, inadequate sleep, a stressful and sedentary lifestyle, and hormonal deficiencies. But the primary underlying cause is decreased energy production.

If you are a man, you can't be healthy and overweight at the same time. If you are a woman, you can be healthy and overweight, but not healthy and obese. This difference between the sexes is because a woman's physiology normally allows her to put on excess weight (up to a certain extent) without it being a consequence of decreased energy production.

Maintaining a healthy level of energy production is critical for maintaining a healthy weight. And, for many people, doing what it takes to keep energy levels high involves the challenge of replacing habits that don't work with new habits that do.

Habits are difficult to break, but it can be done if the will and the desire are strong enough. The good news is, once you develop new habits, they will be just as hard to break as the old ones. And the rewards are great. Healthy weight pays off in terms of a healthier life . . . and a longer life as well.

I would like to offer a *different approach to weight loss* here. It is an approach based on years of guiding my patients who were frustrated by resistant weight problems to a more normal, healthier weight. If this description fits you, the information here can help you reach this critical and elusive health goal.

ARE YOU TOO HEAVY?

Most people can easily tell if they have too much fat simply by looking in the mirror. But a more exact way of assessing obesity is often needed because your fat stores cannot be objectively measured simply by checking your weight.

Your total weight, what you see on the scale, is a mixture of your muscle weight and your fat weight. It is important to know that *muscle weight cancels out the negative effects of fat weight.* Saying that someone has too much body fat is basically the same as saying he/she has too little muscle.

You might wonder how professional football players who have so much obvious fat can still be so quick and powerful. The answer is that underneath the fat, there is a huge amount of muscle, which is not so obvious to the eye.

One of the best ways to determine how much fat and muscle weight you have is by using an electronic technique called bio-impedance measurement. Bio-impedance testing is quick, safe, easy, and readily available in fitness centers and from anti-aging physicians. It involves passing a small level of electrical current through the body. Since muscle and fat each conduct current in different ways, it is possible to determine how much of each is present.

Ideal body-fat measurements are 12–18 percent for men and 18–22 percent for women. Without pulling any punches, let me say that, to the degree your body-fat measurement is greater than this, the odds are that you are unhealthy and will develop diseases that are otherwise completely preventable. As I mentioned earlier, some women (about 30 percent) can even have a body-fat percentage as great as 30 percent and still be healthy, but this can only be determined by Bio-Energy Testing. Unless you have a Bio-Energy Test that proves otherwise, if you are a woman with a fat percentage over 22 percent, you can assume you have a health problem.

HEAVINESS OFFICIALLY DEFINED

The National Institute of Diabetes and Digestive and Kidney Diseases of the National Institutes of Health is the lead federal agency responsible for biomedical research on obesity.

From this resource, we have the following official definitions.

Overweight. An excess amount of body weight that includes muscle, bone, fat, and water.

Obesity. For most people, the term obesity means being very overweight. But obesity specifically refers to an excess amount of body fat. Some people, such as bodybuilders or other athletes with a lot of muscle, can be overweight without being obese. Everyone needs a certain amount of body fat for stored energy, heat insulation, shock absorption, and other functions. As a rule, women have more body fat than men. Most healthcare providers agree that men with more than 25-percent body fat and women with more than 30-percent body fat are obese.

OBESITY = ENERGY DEFICIT

There is no more obvious disorder of energy balance than obesity. And perhaps the most important point regarding obesity and energy production relates to fat metabolism. Let me explain.

Every time anyone eats a meal, the energy from that meal is stored as fat. It doesn't make any difference whether the meal is carbohydrates or fat. Practically speaking, *it all gets stored as fat.* This is how nature designed it.

Humans have evolved over many thousands of years, and our ancestors in the distant past were never quite sure when the next meal was coming. Only recently has the concept of three meals a day become commonplace for many humans. I often tell my patients that people have caveman bodies living in a supermarket world, and it is important to understand that the old physiological process of storing meals as fat has not changed in the last twenty thousand years.

The fat stored from your meal is meant to serve your energy requirements until the next one. But what if your body's ability to produce energy from this stored fat is impaired? *In this case, you will not only gain weight
because you can't burn your stored fat, but you will also produce less energy as
well.* The two go hand in hand. Gaining weight and having low energy are
two sides of the same coin: an inability to burn or metabolize fat. This is
a very common scenario as people get older, and is also why they are often
unable to lose weight.

Except for those individuals who are fat simply from chronic super-siz-
ing, all obese individuals have a serious flaw in the ability to produce energy efficiently. Without measuring energy production and correcting the
underlying disorders of energy production, it becomes almost impossible
to permanently correct obesity.

Here are the facts. Without correcting the underlying energy disorder:

☀ 75 percent of all those who lose weight regain it within three years

☀ 95 percent regain it within ten years

Why were the 5 percent who initially lost weight able to keep it off? No
doubt because they somehow managed to correct the energy-production
deficit that caused their obesity in the first place.

Low energy production causes obesity. And obesity causes low-energy
production.

Many people fall into such a deep hole from this vicious cycle that it
appears impossible for them to escape. What initiates this vicious cycle in
the first place?

TOO MUCH INSULIN

The answer, and the first step towards obesity, involves a loss in energy
production resulting from insulin resistance. Before explaining what this
means, let me take a moment to give you a brief background.

Your DNA, tissues, and organs are made entirely of fat, protein, and
minerals. You consume these raw materials in your food. Your body extracts them from food in the digestive process and, after they are processed
in the liver, uses them as needed.

Carbohydrates are also consumed. But the only use for carbohydrates is
as an energy source. Nothing in your body is made of carbohydrates. Noth-

ing at all. This is why nutritionists will tell you there are *no essential carbo-hydrates*. When a nutritional item is termed *essential*, it means that the nutrient must be present in the diet in order to maintain health, and since the body cannot make the nutrient, it needs to get it from an outside food source. There are essential fats and proteins, but there are no essential car-bohydrates.

Think of carbohydrate foods as treats. Put them in the same general cat-egory as chocolate cake. You don't need to eat chocolate cake to be healthy, but it is nice to have some every now and then. Carbohydrate foods aren't totally useless, however. Your body extracts vitamins and minerals from many of these foods. And assuming it has not been processed out (as in refined flours and grains), the fiber contained in the carbohydrates is used by the body as roughage to promote elimination of waste products. But the complete truth is that the major ingredients in carbohydrate foods are sugars, and sugars are not essential to anything.

The absorbed sugars extracted from the carbohydrates represent a raw material for energy production. That's all. And the reality is, the body can make all the energy it needs from fat alone. So it doesn't need any dietary sugar. It's not essential to your health.

When carbohydrates are consumed, the body does one or two things with the extracted sugars—it burns them for energy, or stores them as fat. The decision whether to burn or store is primarily determined by hor-mones. And the most important hormone in this scenario is insulin, which is secreted by the pancreas according to how much carbohydrate is in your diet.

The connection between carbohydrate consumption and obesity is this: *The more carbohydrates you eat, the more insulin the pancreas makes. And the presence of too much insulin is a primary cause of obesity because insulin diverts ingested carbohydrates to fat storage and away from energy production.* So it is easy to see why excess insulin creates a low energy state combined with increased body fat. And here's the rest of the story.

Besides diverting carbohydrates to fat storage, the other function of insu-lin is to prevent the breakdown and utilization of stored fat. And because insulin prevents fat utilization, in a state of insulin excess, your body will have to get an increasing amount of your energy from your glycogen (car-bohydrate) stores.

The significant difference between glycogen and fat stores is that the body can only store a very small amount of glycogen. Only enough to provide energy for one or two hours. But by comparison, fat stores can provide energy for days and even weeks. So, in a state of insulin excess, your body will start to produce less and less energy from fat, and more and more energy from glycogen.

This means two things.

1. Only a few hours after eating, your glycogen stores will become depleted, and you will begin to run out of energy. This is a state known as hypoglycemia, or low blood sugar.

2. You will have a persistent craving for carbohydrates to replenish the exhausted glycogen stores.

THE INSULIN/CARBOHYDRATE VICIOUS CYCLE

Too many carbohydrates in your diet sets up a vicious cycle. It stimulates the body to make more insulin. The more insulin you make, the more difficult it is for your body to access fat for energy, and so the more your body will rely on your glycogen stores. The more you use up your glycogen stores, the more you need to eat carbohydrates to replenish them. Ad infinitum.

The nasty effects of this cycle stem from the resulting hypoglycemia and decreased energy production. They include anxiety, depression, fatigue, headaches, insomnia, and lack of endurance. Another very common effect is a persistent weight gain—weight you will absolutely not be able to lose, even when you exercise and limit caloric intake. Let me repeat. In a state of insulin excess, *you will not be able to lose weight, even if you exercise and limit calories until you are blue in the face.*

The result of this insulin/carbohydrate vicious cycle is a condition called insulin resistance. Insulin resistance refers to the decreased ability of the body's cells to respond to insulin, hence they are described as being resistant to the hormone. Insulin resistance occurs when there is a decrease in energy production combined with excessive carbohydrate intake.

How do you know if you eating too many carbohydrates? One sign is weight gain, but another way to find out is through Bio-Energy Testing. If you are overindulging in carbohydrates, the test will show this as an abnormally low C-Factor. (*See* Chapter 7, Carbohydrate Factor.)

ENLARGED FAT CELLS/INSULIN RESISTANCE VICIOUS CYCLE

When the body's cells become resistant to insulin, the pancreas responds by making more insulin, and another vicious cycle is created. As the insulin resistance continues over years, the pancreas keeps pumping out ever-increasing amounts of insulin to overcome it. Ultimately a state of chronic insulin excess develops, which continuously blocks the utilization of fat stores for energy production. This, in turn, results in the low-energy production and excessive fat stores that cause obesity.

As this situation continues, the fat cells themselves become progressively larger (the fat cells become fatter). They expand to such an extent that the insulin-receptor sites on the membranes become stretched and distorted, and are then unable to properly respond to insulin. In other words, these engorged fat cells become more resistant to insulin, which acts to further increase the already elevated insulin levels.

HOW WEIGHT GAIN CAUSES LOW ENERGY

There's still more to this drama of vicious cycles. You've seen how low-energy production causes weight gain. Now look at the opposite—how weight gain causes low energy. I personally believe that the low-energy state comes first, but this is pretty much a moot point. The reality is, when most people become concerned about their weight, both factors are in full force—low-energy production and obesity.

Weight gain results in low-energy production in several known ways. The first is, since it is always associated with decreased muscle, it results in a decreased metabolic rate. This is because muscle tissue is so metabolically active that when it becomes depleted the metabolic rate falls. Metabolic rate refers to how many calories a body burns when it is at rest. Thus, metabolic rate is used as a measurement of basic energy production. A low metabolic rate is measured by Bio-Energy Testing as an abnormally low M-Factor. (*See* Chapter 7, Metabolic Factor.)

Second, weight gain causes a variety of sleep disturbances. These disturbances are often manifested by snoring and daytime sleepiness, but are frequently present without symptoms and often can only be detected in a sleep lab. A very common problem with weight gain is that it interferes with the body's ability to enter into what is known as the *slow-wave* stage of sleep. Since the majority of growth-hormone production occurs during slow-wave sleep, this leads to a deficiency of growth hormone. The most common consequence of growth-hormone deficiency is a decrease in muscle mass and an increase in fat mass.

Third, the sleep disturbances associated with weight gain create more insulin resistance. How this occurs is still unknown, but the fact that it happens is well-documented.

Fourth, weight gain causes an excess of estrogens. This is because fat cells metabolically increase estrogens in the body, independent of ovarian and adrenal-gland production. In excess, estrogens suppress the mitochondria, resulting in a significant reduction in the metabolic rate. Estrogens also cause the body to retain and increase fat stores.

NOTE TO MEN

Excess estrogens also affect you because you produce estrogens in the adrenal glands, and as you age, a greater proportion of your testosterone gets converted to estrogen. This not only causes fat gain, but can also contribute to prostate enlargement and prostate cancer.

Fifth, overweight people quite naturally engage in less physical activity. How much do you think you would you like to go jogging or play basketball if you were twenty to thirty pounds overweight? A sedentary lifestyle translates to a lower metabolic rate. Often, overweight individuals are exercise intolerant—they can easily slip into anaerobic-energy production, which makes exercising very difficult. This is where Bio-Energy Testing can be so helpful. It can pinpoint the exact exercise zones for maximum fat burning and metabolism even in obese people.

OTHER WEIGHT-CONTROL AGGRAVATORS

The factors already discussed form the basis for most of the weight-control problems for overweight individuals. But there are still several others that can confound a weight-loss effort.

One is sunlight deficiency. Several studies examining the effects of sunlight deficiency have demonstrated a significant association with a lowered metabolic rate in both animals and humans. This occurs as a result of hormonal deficiencies associated with a lack of sunlight, plus other as-yet-unidentified effects of sunlight on the metabolism.

Stress is another cause of decreased metabolism. In many individuals, prolonged stress decreases the metabolic rate through its negative impact on the output of the adrenal glands. This leads to low blood sugar, low energy production, and weight gain.

Inadequate water intake also depresses the metabolism. And dehydration can lead to overeating because it can cause the feeling of hunger. Drinking water often reduces feelings of hunger.

Insomnia and lack of adequate rest can lower the metabolic rate as well. And then there is the issue of emotional eating. In our overfed society, much of what we consider hunger can have more to do with emotions than with real physical need. I believe that everyone, skinny and fat alike, has an eating disorder to some extent. Periodic fasting (*see* Chapter 12, Secret Five) can help you identify how much of a reality this might be for you.

Training yourself to be comfortable and relaxed when you are hungry is a major step towards solving the problem of emotional eating. An invaluable technique to help you develop this strength is to fast once a week, and use the breath-meditation exercise when you feel hungry. This won't lessen your feeling of hunger, but it will help you control all the emotions that hunger stirs up.

METABOLIC WEIGHT LOSS

If you have a serious weight problem, you now know the possible reasons for it. What's next is to lose the weight. Anybody can lose weight. There are hundreds of books that will tell you how to do this. That part is easy. What's hard is keeping the weight off. And to do that you must normalize your energy production. You must make that a primary goal.

HOW MUCH FAT DO YOU LOSE WHILE YOU'RE SLEEPING?

Your energy-production level at rest, when you are sleeping, is referred to as your basal metabolism. A tenet of the Energy-Deficit Theory of aging is that no matter what age you are, or what genetics you've been dealt, your basal metabolism should ideally be maintained at youthful levels. From the perspective of weight gain, basal metabolism can best be described as that measurement which determines how much fat you burn while you are sleeping.

It has often been said that the only way to really become rich is to make money while you are sleeping. I can promise you it is also true that the only way you can control your weight is to lose fat while you are sleeping. And the only way to do this is to optimize your metabolism.

The process of optimizing your metabolism literally involves each and every one of the secrets I've developed in this book. Often the most crucial aspects of optimizing the metabolism are a reduction in dietary carbohydrates to what is right for your genetics, combined with weightlifting, exercising at your fat-burning rate, adequate sleep, and natural hormone replacement. Having an optimal metabolism forms the basis of what I refer to as permanent metabolic weight loss.

YOU'RE NOT TOO FAT—YOU'RE TOO WEAK

The more I have researched the dynamics of what makes some people thin and others fat, the more I have begun to appreciate the importance of muscle mass. I am convinced that the low metabolism consistently seen in almost every overweight person is to a large extent due to decreased muscle mass.

I am so convinced of this, I tell my patients that for permanent weight control, it is much more important to gain muscle than lose fat. Their decrease in muscle mass is the result of frequent dieting, genetics, hormonal imbalances, aging, and lack of proper exercise. Careful attention to all these factors is critical to success. Any weight-loss program that doesn't seriously focus on increasing muscle mass is doomed to failure.

HOW TO INCREASE YOUR ENERGY
AND LOSE YOUR FAT PERMANENTLY

Following the seven steps outlined here can help you achieve these goals.

Step 1—Diagnosing Insulin Resistance

Do you have insulin resistance that is contributing to excess weight in your body? The most reliable way I have found to assess the presence and degree of insulin resistance is with Bio-Energy Testing.

Another easy way to determine insulin resistance is simply to check a fasting insulin blood level. The normal range for fasting insulin in the United States is 5–25 micro units per milliliter (uiu/mL), but any values greater than 10 uiu/mL mean that insulin resistance is present. This so-called normal range for fasting insulin levels only serves to demonstrate how common insulin resistance is because it means that more than half the *healthy* people in the United States have significant insulin resistance.

Is it just coincidental that half the population in the United States is insulin resistant and half the population is overweight? I don't think so. I believe it just indicates that insulin resistance is the cause of weight gain in an overwhelming number of people. Insulin levels need to be brought down below a minimum of 10 uiu/mL before successful weight loss can occur.

An additional, sensitive way to make the diagnosis is with a fasting blood-lipid test. Since insulin acts to divert foods to fat, it causes an elevation of fats in the blood. An elevation in cholesterol and triglycerides alerts me to the possibility of excess insulin. An elevation of a fraction of triglycerides known as VLDL (very low-density lipoprotein) is a particularly strong indicator.

Step 2—Addressing Insulin Resistance

Dietary carbohydrates stimulate the release of insulin. So it would seem that the most immediate and effective way to reduce the tide of insulin in the body is to reduce carbohydrate consumption. And indeed, in milder cases this is the solution.

Carbohydrates stimulate the release of insulin in everyone. However, some people release much more insulin than normal after a carbohydrate meal. This condition is referred to as a carbohydrate sensitivity. If you are carbohydrate-sensitive, you should be very careful not to eat more carbohydrates than your body can handle.

How much should you cut back on carbohydrate consumption? That varies greatly from person to person. A useful guide is to keep cutting carbohydrates back until the C-Factor measurement on Bio-Energy Testing is over 90 (*see* Chapter 7), and the fasting insulin is less than 10 uiu/mL. In some cases, almost all dietary carbohydrate must be eliminated in order to achieve these goals.

Using the Glycemic Index

Researchers have discovered that certain carbohydrates stimulate the release of more insulin than others. This observation has led to a ranking of carbohydrates according to their insulin effect. This list is known as the glycemic index, and here is how it works.

When carbohydrates are designated with a high-glycemic rating, this means they cause the release of elevated levels of insulin. Middle- and low-glycemic carbohydrates release progressively less insulin.

Carbohydrate-sensitive individuals should decrease the consumption of carbohydrates in general, but should particularly avoid foods that have a high-glycemic rating. Limited amounts of low- or middle-glycemic carbohydrates may be permitted on an individual basis.

THE GLYCEMIC INDEX

High Glycemic

1. Bread (white), cookies, crackers, pancakes, pastry, pretzels, and most flour products, with the exception of pasta.

2. Barley, cold breakfast cereals (including muesli), chips, cooked cereals (except slow-cooked oatmeal), corn, millet, and rice (white).

3. Bananas, mangoes, melons, papayas, pineapples, pumpkins, and raisins.

4. All sweets. This means anything that tastes sweet, including barley malt, corn syrup, fruit juices, high-fructose corn syrup, honey, maltodextrin, maltose, maple syrup, molasses, and sugar. Always check ingredient labels for sugars. Anything that ends in the suffix **ose** is a sugar. The exceptions in the sweet category are pure fructose and the herb stevia.

5. All root vegetables, with the exception of yams. This includes beets, carrots, potatoes, and sweet potatoes.

6. Beer and wine (even low-alcohol). All liquor other than vodka and gin.

Middle Glycemic

1. Apples, oranges, peaches, pears, and plums.

2. Ezekial brand bread (made from grain sprouts rather than the grain itself) high-protein pasta, and yams.

3. Garbanzo beans, kidney beans (canned), navy beans, peas, and pinto beans.

4. Gin and vodka

Low Glycemic

1. Black-eyed peas, chick peas, kidney beans, lentils, and lima beans.

2. Soybeans and soy products, such as miso, soy protein, tempeh, and tofu. Be aware that soy products will often contain sugar.

3. Apricots, berries, cherries, grapefruits, grapes, milk, and nuts.

4. Slow-cooked oatmeal and 100-percent whole grain rye bread.

5. Fructose. This is the only low-glycemic sugar. It is quite sweet.

Step 3—Diet Concerns

Besides monitoring your intake of carbohydrates, there are three other dietary considerations that must be addressed.

☀ The first relates to total calories. In order to lose weight, total calories must be carefully restricted. That means restricted enough to result in fat loss, but not enough to cause muscle loss. Bio-Energy Testing is so helpful because the correct caloric intake is extremely important and very individual. Through it you can determine your basal metabolic rate (BMR). Increase this number by 10 percent and that's the number of calories you should eat per day to lose weight. Be very careful about using charts, formulas, or graphs to determine your basal metabolic rate. These are almost always off by as much as 400–800 calories. If you don't have access to Bio-Energy Testing, you will just have to guess.

☀ The second key consideration is to avoid hydrogenated oils, also known as trans fats. These man-made oils become incorporated into the membranes of every cell in your body and interfere with many of the essential functions of the cell. Their negative effect may well be a major contributor in the development of insulin resistance. Hydrogenated oils are commonly found in baked goods, margarine, mayonnaise, and almost any packaged convenience food. The health warnings on these have now been sounded far and wide, and they have been replaced in many products, but they are still out there and are still dangerous.

☀ The third consideration is to learn to be comfortable with hunger. When you are hungry, it indicates that your glycogen stores are exhausted, and that you are meeting your energy requirements from your fat reserves, which is exactly what losing fat is all about. If you feel hungry between meals, just relax. It's absolutely OK to be hungry. In many cases it is even necessary in order to be successful. Don't immediately run to the cookie jar or pull out a 30–30–40 bar from your desk drawer. Drink a glass of water and get on with your day. You will often find that hunger lessens as you get over the hump and begin to access your fat stores better. Please don't yield to hunger. The majority of the time people feel hunger, it's for emotional reasons, anyway.

Step 4—Supplements

Nutritional deficiencies are often lurking behind insulin resistance. For people who are genetically susceptible to insulin resistance, missing or deficient nutrients cannot be adequately supplied by diet alone. They must be provided through supplements that, in order to be effective, must be taken in the correct form and dosage. That is why I developed Quick-Start, a powerful nutritional formula in powder form that contains the necessary nutrients in their proper potency (*see* Appendix A for ingredients list). QuickStart is a key element for my patients with stubborn weight problems.

In addition to this formula, I also recommend flax oil or, better yet, Super Fat, and the amino acid L-carnitine to help bring down elevated insulin levels. One scoop of QuickStart is blended with one tablespoon of flax oil or Super Fat (see page 185 for further suggestions). This smoothie is taken in the morning and afternoon.

Patients with mild insulin resistance are usually able to resolve the problem by avoiding the high-glycemic carbohydrates, taking the supplements, and exercising regularly. Obese individuals may require the additional help of the following specialized supplements.

Coenzyme Q_{10}

This vitaminlike substance, produced naturally in the body, is a key ingredient in cellular energy production. It becomes depleted with age, or as a result of poor diet or taking cholesterol-lowering drugs. Not surprisingly, it is often deficient in overweight people. If your fasting-blood CoQ_{10} level is below 1.5 mg/L, you should supplement with enough of this enzyme to reach this minimum level. Typical doses are in the range of 30–100 milligrams per day.

Alpha lipoic acid

Alpha-lipoic acid, a first-line antioxidant in the body, also becomes depleted as people age. The decline is even more marked in individuals with insulin resistance. Alpha-lipoic acid is an essential nutrient for fat metabolism. The recommended dose is 100–200 milligrams daily.

Conjugated linoleic acid (CLA)

There are several studies in both humans and animals verifying the fat-metabolizing effect of conjugated linoleic acid (CLA), a naturally occurring oil amply contained in animal fats. Strict vegetarians tend to be particularly low in this oil. CLA, at doses ranging from 1,000–2,000 milligrams three times a day, helps lower the insulin level.

Growth-hormone stimulators

The amino acids L-lysine and L-glutamine cause the body to produce extra growth hormone. This is especially useful in a weight-management program because overweight people are often deficient in growth hormone. Growth hormone is *the* key hormone in maintaining an optimal fat-to-muscle ratio, so you can see how important it is for weight control.

Take 3,000 mg of L-lysine on an empty stomach when you first wake up in the morning. Take 2,000 mg of L-glutamine on an empty stomach at bedtime.

Step 5—Natural Hormone Replacement

The hormone deficiencies most often responsible for the low-energy production causing weight gain are progesterone (in women), testosterone (in women and men), the adrenal and thyroid hormones, and growth hormone.

Successful long-term weight control very often requires replacement of these hormones on an individually-tailored basis. Since I believe a weight-loss program may not succeed without such replacement, I suggest consulting a physician specializing in anti-aging medicine who is experienced in working with natural hormones.

Step 6—Correct Exercise

Two very effective exercise methods for weight control are FBR training and circuit training.

FBR training

When you exercise at a heart rate equal to your fat-burning rate (FBR), your body is burning fat as fast as it can. As the exertion level increases beyond this point, the proportion of energy produced from fat metabolism actually decreases until you reach a point at which you don't burn any fat at all. Unfortunately, due to their energy-production deficit and insulin irregularity, overweight people usually spend all their exercise time at this latter level. Instead of burning fat, they are only burning their limited supply of glycogen.

My new patients who are overweight tell me that no matter how hard they exercise, they can't lose weight. No wonder. They just haven't learned the mechanics of their current state of physiology.

Proper exercise for fat loss means spending more time at a lower level of exertion. This means a minimum of thirty to forty-five minutes a day exercising at the FBR. For individuals with an aversion to exercise, this is good news indeed. Exercising at this level is very comfortable. So comfortable, in fact, that you could be exercising at this rate while talking on the

---

THE SHALLENBERGER BLUE PLATE SPECIAL

Food, Supplements, and Liquid for a More Streamlined You

Carefully follow the instructions below. They work. In almost all cases, this approach will lead to one to two pounds of fat loss per week.

FOOD

Breakfast: One scoop of QuickStart blended with one teaspoon of flax oil or Super Fat.
Eggs, meats (meats include fish, poultry, and red meat), and regular, unsweetened yogurt are optional.

Lunch: Salad with dressing, cheese, and meats, or stir-fried vegetables with meat.

Dinner: Meats, vegetables, salad, beans.

Snacks: A little of what you had the last meal.

Desserts: One piece of whole, fresh fruit from the middle- or low-glycemic list eaten right after dinner.

Exceptions: Two meals per week with rice, bread, or soy-based pasta.

General eating guidelines: Eat slowly and be relaxed. Chew your food well. Enjoy your meals. Eat only what you need. Feel free to skip meals. Salt and spices are unlimited. Cream may be used in moderation. You may use one tablespoon

phone, and the person you are talking to would never guess you were exercising at all.

Exercising at your FBR, for example on a treadmill or stationary bicycle, is the perfect kind of exercise to do while watching TV or reading. Your FBR can be exactly determined with Bio-Energy Testing. You can fairly accurately guess it by noting what your heart rate is at an exercise level where you are just starting to feel slightly out of breath.

Circuit training

Circuit training consists of a particular kind of weight training, also known as resistance training. If you are not familiar with weight training, you will definitely need to work with someone experienced, such as a personal

---

of fructose or xylitol a day as a sweetener. Do not eat anything for at least three hours before bedtime.

DRINKS

Water is your preferred beverage. (See Chapter 8, Secret One, for how much to drink.)

Definitely limit your diet sodas. One per day, if at all.

Four 4-ounce cups of coffee or green tea per day are permitted.

Herbal tea is unlimited.

No fruit juice.

SUPPLEMENTS

Immediately after you wake up, take 2 grams of L-lysine with a glass of water. Wait at least forty-five minutes before eating.

As noted above, take QuickStart in the morning.

Take 2,000 milligrams of conjugated linoleic acid (CLA) three times per day.

Take 100 milligrams of coenzymeQ_{10}, 1 gram of L-carnitine, and 100 milligrams of alpha-lipoic acid two times per day.

Take another scoop of QuickStart blended with one teaspoon of flax oil or Super Fat around 3 or 4 PM.

Take 2 grams of L-glutamine at bedtime.

LAURIE'S JOURNEY TO LOOKING AND FEELING GREAT

When I first saw Laurie, she was forty-three-years old and weighed 220 pounds. Most of her weight gain had occurred during the previous nine years, a prolonged period of marital and job stress. During this time she exercised only sporadically. She had gone on several diets, lost twenty or thirty pounds on them, but soon put the weight back. Now, she complained, "I can't seem to lose weight no matter what I do."

Sound familiar?

Before her weight explosion, Laurie had weighed 150 pounds and had felt and looked great at that weight. But now, at 220, her body-fat percentage was almost 50 percent—half of her, 110 pounds, was fat. The other 110 pounds reflected her lean body mass, which essentially equates to her muscle mass. Assuming she had a healthy body-fat percentage of 22 percent before she gained all the weight, her fat would have been 30 pounds, and her muscle mass 120 pounds.

So what was her problem? Was it that she gained eighty pounds of fat, or that she lost ten pounds of muscle mass? The answer is that the lost ten pounds of muscle is actually more of a contributing factor to her obesity than the gained eighty pounds of fat. This is because muscle tissue is extremely active metabolically, and burns a significant amount of fat calories even while sleeping. The more muscle mass you have, reflected by a greater lean-body-mass percentage, the greater your daily fat-calorie expenditure will be. Laurie's ten-pound decrease in muscle mass was easily enough of a loss to prevent her from successfully burning her fat stores.

Every time Laurie embarked on a weight-loss plan, she lost much more than she bargained for. Each time she indeed did lose weight, but the lost weight included muscle loss. This is because weight-loss plans do not focus on the real problem with weight gain, a decrease in energy production. In fact, weight-loss programs only aggravate the situation because, in the absence of proper metabolic management, calorie restriction causes the body to lower its metabolic rate even more.

The only way to lose **just** fat and no muscle is by combining calorie restriction with proper exercise, sleep, sunlight, supplementation, and hormonal replacement if it is needed.

Laurie's muscle loss also increased her insulin resistance. This is because muscle cells have an enormous number of insulin receptors. Loss of muscle mass, therefore, results in a loss of total body-insulin receptors, in turn causing elevated insulin levels.

Because her muscle loss caused her metabolism to decrease and her insulin resistance to increase, Laurie ultimately regained all the fat she had lost—and then some. She gained back the fat, but unfortunately not the muscle. Over the years, this yo-yo effect caused her to lose enough muscle to put her in a hole she could not climb out of.

But it wasn't just a lack of exercise and repeated dieting that caused her problems. It was also the fact that she had gone from being thirty-four to forty-three-years-old, and had developed the hormonal deficiencies that come with getting older. Since hormones play such an important role in maintaining muscles, a common side effect with deficiencies is a loss of muscle mass. All these elements fit into the equation of solving Laurie's weight problem.

Hormone Replacement and Correct Exercise

The first thing we did was to give Laurie a Bio-Energy Test. (Chapter 7 will tell you all you need to know about this important advance in weight management.) The results provided the necessary information to customize a personal and effective program for this unhappy woman.

Bio-Energy Testing indicated that Laurie had low-thyroid activity, known as hypothyroidism. As with so many cases of hypothyroidism, her blood testing was in range; only her Bio-Energy Testing was sensitive enough to diagnose the problem. The primary effect of low-thyroid function is to lower the metabolic rate. Her Bio-Energy Testing revealed that her metabolic rate was only 76 percent of optimal. Based on this reading, I prescribed enough thyroid hormones to return her metabolic rate to normal.

Laurie's Bio-Energy Testing also determined her FBR. I explained to her that she needed to begin exercising three times a week for thirty minutes at her FBR. Another three days a week I had her performing circuit training. Our in-house clinic trainer taught her how to do this. Then, every six to eight weeks she would meet with the trainer to update her progress, and alter her exercise protocol as needed.

Next, her Bio-Energy Testing revealed a C-Factor of 50. As you will see in Chapter 7, this meant that her consumption of carbohydrates was completely suppressing her fat metabolism. Instead of burning fat for energy, her body was living off carbohydrates. Clearly she was eating way too many carbohydrates, and was already insulin resistant. I told her that if she wanted to permanently cure her weight problem, the carbohydrates were going to have to go.

Finally, hormone testing revealed she was in a state of relative estrogen excess, and that her DHEA was depleted. This did not surprise me. As an anabolic hormone, DHEA is very much involved in the production of muscle tissue, and it is also extremely valuable in correcting insulin resistance.

To overcome these imbalances, I prescribed a DHEA supplement and a topical progesterone cream for her estrogen excess. All her hormone levels were regularly rechecked to ensure that she was being administered the correct doses for her individual needs. (See Chapter 15, Secret Eight, on bio-identical hormone replacement.)

Laurie was determined to beat her weight problem. So, armed with new information and several natural prescriptions, she set off to remake herself. And she succeeded. Within a year she had lost fifty-five pounds of fat. More importantly, through her exercise program, she had **gained** five pounds of muscle.

As an additional reward for her tenacity, Laurie no longer needed to adhere so strictly to carbohydrate avoidance because her fat loss, muscle gain, and hormonal replacement had completely eliminated her insulin resistance. She had literally made her body over. Ironically however, Laurie was like so many of my patients who are addicted to carbohydrates. Once she had experienced what these non-essential treat foods were doing to her, she no longer considered them a treat and she completely lost her desire for them.

Now, more than eleven years later, she still has her former figure back and continues to maintain her desired weight simply by following the guidelines I recommend in this book.

Laurie's case is not exceptional. In fact, it's typical. When energy production is normalized, it is possible for any overweight individual to achieve—and maintain—a permanent and healthy weight level.

---

trainer, to get you started and periodically check up on how you're doing. The circuit training I have found most useful is performed within the following specific parameters.

1. The resistance training must exercise the muscles of the arms, chest, back, abdomen and, most importantly, the legs. This would include arm curls, military presses, bench presses, pull ups, abdominal crunches, and squats or lunges.

2. The exercises are performed in 3–4 sets of 25 repetitions.

3. The sets are repeated continuously for 35–40 minutes.

4. At the end of each set, wait until your heart rate has dropped to your FBR before starting the next set.

Additional pointers

Rome wasn't built in a day. Neither will you get in shape the first day, or maybe even the first month. In fact, when you first start exercising, you probably will not be able to do half as much as you would like. Just be patient. It will all come around as you continue forward and get in progressively better shape.

Perform the FBR training three days a week, and the circuit training three days a week. Take one day a week off to rest and be lazy. A successful program will usually result in losing anywhere from ten to fifteen pounds the first few weeks. Most of this is water loss so don't get too excited. After this period, expect to lose about one to two pounds of weight per week. When you have lost the weight, you will only need to exercise for thirty minutes three times a week to maintain your health and optimum energy production.

Step 7—Sleep, Sunlight, and Water

I can't emphasize strongly enough the importance of adequate rest in order for your body to generate good energy. Be sure to get in seven or eight hours of quality sleep on most nights—*this often means disciplining yourself to go to bed earlier.*

And while I am in emphasis mode, I should also remind you about getting enough sunlight and drinking enough water. Getting enough sleep, sunlight, and water is free, at least so far. But even though they cost you nothing, please don't think they are any less important than the other things we have been discussing. It may not be obvious, but sleep, sunlight, and water are all important for helping you with your weight problem and putting you on the fast track to be bursting with energy.

My Recommendations to You

⁂ Carefully follow the food and supplement instructions outlined.

⁂ Obtain a weight-composition analysis through bio-impedance testing, available at most health spas. The ideal body-fat percentages are 18–22 percent for women and 12–18 percent for men. If your measurements are in line, follow my recommendations to avoid developing a weight problem.

⁂ If your body-fat percentage is above these levels, you have a weight problem that needs to be resolved. The most efficient way to do that is to obtain Bio-Energy Testing. (*See* Chapter 7 for the details.) The test will provide you with your particular exercise zones, and accurately measure your metabolism and fat burning capacity.

✳ Regardless of what blood tests show, if your metabolism is below normal, you may very likely need thyroid-hormone replacement in order to be successful. If your physician isn't familiar with physiological hormone replacement and won't prescribe thyroid replacement unless the blood tests are out of the normal range, I suggest finding another doctor who can help you. For a referral, contact either the American College for the Advancement of Medicine at 949-309-3520 (www.acam.org) or the American Academy of Anti-Aging Medicine at 773-528-1000 (www.worldhealth.net).

✳ Exercise three days a week for thirty to forty-five minutes at your FBR. Spend another three days with thirty-five to forty minutes of circuit training. I very strongly recommend that you work with a personal trainer to help you achieve your goals.

✳ Obtain a Bio-Energy Testing recheck after every twenty-five to thirty pounds of fat loss. The reason is that energy measurements will improve as weight comes off, and the program will have to be adjusted accordingly.

✳ As you lose weight, you can also monitor progress from time to time with additional bio-impedance analysis. A correct exercise program will result in putting on muscle weight even as you lose fat weight, so your overall weight may not reflect your net fat loss, and the best way to follow your results is by bio-impedance analysis. You can also measure your waist, thighs, and hips, and take a good look in the mirror as you take off the weight and tone yourself up.

✳ The hormones intimately involved with weight management are DHEA, estrogen, growth hormone, progesterone, testosterone, and the thyroid hormones. Unless your physician has been trained in *natural* hormone replacement, you will need a specialist in this field. Contact the organizations listed for a referral.

✳ Practice regular breath meditation, and be sure to get plenty of water and a full night's sleep. Oh, and don't forget about sunlight.

6

Energy and Detoxification

As you've watched friends and relatives over the years, you've no doubt wondered why some people age so much more rapidly than others. The basic reason is that those who age faster have less ability to generate adequate levels of energy.

Genetics aside, toxicity is one of the greatest factors influencing the age-related decrease in energy production. By toxicity, I mean the progressive accumulation of harmful substances, referred to as toxins, in the cells and tissues of the body.

Toxins can come from the environment in the form of chemicals, cigarettes, food additives, heavy metals, and pharmaceutical drugs, but surprisingly, the overwhelming source of toxicity is the body itself. Each and every cell in the body takes in oxygen and nutrients, and from these substances produces energy *and* waste products. The wastes materialize in the form of organic acids. They are very toxic, and must be moved out of the system in order to maintain health. Other sources of toxicity in the body include the bowels, the mouth, and the sinuses.

Regardless of the source, the important thing to know is that toxins decrease cellular-energy production. Since the very tissues and organs that are responsible for the treatment and removal of bodily toxins require substantial energy production themselves, a vicious cycle is created, resulting in a persistent decline in energy production as people become older.

All the secrets I'll be sharing with you in Part Two relate to detoxification and improving your energy level. But before I begin giving you practical how-to information, I want to discuss toxicity and detoxification (toxin removal).

YOUR INTERNAL SEWER

It's not a very pleasant scene down in the lower intestine after the remnants of food have passed through the digestive and absorption processes. Basically, you're looking at an internal sewer, teeming with bacterial and fungal life, putrefied matter, incompletely digested foods, dyes, pesticides, preservatives, and probably a fair share of parasites.

Your body deals with this mess in a number of ways. First and foremost, more than 90 percent of your immune-system activity occurs in the intestinal tract where the immune cells are constantly battling foreign invaders and toxins. To do the job well, this activity requires a huge amount of energy. But, as good as the immune system is, it can't prevent all the bowel's toxins from finding their way into the bloodstream.

Fortunately, before it enters the general circulation, the blood that circulates in the intestines, and picks up all the nutrients and toxins, passes through the liver where the toxins are filtered out. I say fortunately because, if the liver was not there to do this job, within a matter of hours you would die from your own internal toxins—that's how important the liver is to your health.

The liver also requires an enormous amount of energy production to accomplish its critical janitorial services. As long as it functions optimally, it can effectively protect the rest of the body from toxicity, but as illness and the aging process erode this energy production, liver function diminishes. As a result, more toxic materials, many of them carcinogenic, are able to get through the liver and into the general circulation.

ORAL TOXINS

Dr. Gary Verigin is a friend and internationally respected biological dentist (a biological dentist is one who appreciates and understands how dramatically your dental health affects your overall health). Dr. Verigin told me long ago, "the routine use in dentistry of silver amalgam fillings is a major source of toxicity in the human body." My experience with my patients' various health disorders has confirmed this statement.

Since the late 1800s, dentists have been using silver amalgam fillings as a preferred treatment for cavities. Many years ago, I was shocked to learn that 50 percent of these amalgams are comprised of mercury, an extremely toxic heavy metal. An average amalgam filling contains about 780 milligrams of mercury, enough to exceed the U.S. Environmental Protection Agency's non-dietary mercury-intake standard for 100 years.

Dentists have always thought that once amalgam fillings were mixed and put in place, the mercury was somehow locked in. Some years ago, however, researchers learned this is *not* the case. They revealed that mercury vapor is *continuously* released in the mouth by the activity of brushing, chewing, and drinking hot liquids, constantly exposing people with silver amalgams to mercury every day.

Mercury is more toxic than arsenic, cadmium, or lead. Other than fluoride, it is the most toxic of all naturally occurring substances. Organic mercury, called methyl mercury, and the inorganic form found in the vapor from amalgams are the most toxic forms. There is no known non-toxic level for mercury vapor.

The vapor easily enters the body, where levels of mercury build up with time. *Mercury is a potent suppressor of mitochondrial activity,* and it damages brain and nerve tissue, the adrenal, pituitary, and thyroid glands, the heart and lungs, as well as hormones and enzymes.

Additional research indicates that mercury collects in the body's tissues, suppresses the immune system, forms mutated strains of fungi and bacteria, and contributes to allergies and auto-immune disorders, such as lupus, multiple sclerosis, and rheumatoid arthritis.

Mercury penetrates the placental membrane easily and has been found to damage the brain and nervous system of unborn babies. For that reason, the American Dental Association has recommended that silver amalgam fillings not be placed in the mouths of pregnant women. What is ignored is the effect of the mercury fillings already in place in these women.

Mercury depletes the immune system. In one study, immune helper cells, which regulate immune-system operations, were significantly suppressed in every person tested until their silver amalgams were removed. Furthermore, these same immune cells were determined to be almost immediately suppressed when silver amalgams were placed in the mouths of those previously without them. Other studies have revealed that the ingested mercury released from silver amalgam fillings causes the yeast organisms commonly found in the intestines to become resistant to the normal function of the immune system.

The federal Occupational Safety and Health Administration (OSHA) and the Environmental Protection Agency (EPA) have declared that left-over scrap dental amalgam is a toxic hazard to dental personnel, to the dental office, and to the environment. Ironically, these agencies require very rigid protocols for the handling and disposal of the exact same dental material that is placed in our mouths.

Chronic mercury poisoning can affect all the body tissues and can mimic many common diseases. Many people recover from diseases after the fillings are removed, and the residual mercury is chelated (chemically removed) from the body.

It is important to note that, because of genetic susceptibility, some individuals are very sensitive to certain toxins, whereas others are much less sensitive. This is why the various side effects from medications only happen to certain people—not to everyone. Mainstream medicine tends to downplay the effects of environmental toxicity because it often only affects those who are sensitive and leaves the rest of us alone. Many people who develop chronic environmental poisoning, such as that stemming from mercury dental fillings, are told it is all in their heads because they are the only ones affected. Perhaps, in some cases, this is true, but I have seen many patients over the past thirty-five years who get much better when those fillings are removed, and they are placed on an aggressive detoxification program. The following are the most prevalent signs and symptoms of chronic mercury poisoning.

※ Cardiovascular effects—Alterations in blood pressure, feeble and irregular pulse, irregular heartbeat, pain and pressure in the chest.

※ Neurological effects—Coordination difficulties, chronic or frequent headaches, dizziness, speech difficulties, tremors.

※ Psychological effects—Anxiety, depression, fits of anger, irritability, loss of self-confidence, loss of self-control, memory loss, nervousness, shyness, or timidity.

※ Respiratory effects—Emphysema, persistent cough, shallow and irregular respiration.

※ Other effects—Abdominal cramps, allergies, anemia, bleeding gums, bone loss, cold and clammy skin, colitis, diarrhea, edema, excessive perspiration, excessive salivation, fatigue, foul breath, joint pains, loosening of teeth, metallic taste in mouth, muscle weakness, and sub-normal temperature.

CHRONIC SINUS INFECTIONS—JUST WATCH TV

The inflammation stemming from allergies and chronic sinus infections is a very common source of toxicity. You just have to watch TV and count the advertisements for sinus medication to know this is really a big problem.

Allergies to foods and inhalants are the cause. Interestingly enough, as people age, allergies tend to disappear. This is because allergies are an over-reaction of the immune system. The immune system requires a huge amount of energy to operate, and as people grow older and energy production declines, immunity declines as well, resulting in a decreased incidence of allergies. Nevertheless, long before the allergies have gone away, chronic sinus infections have often taken root, and a depressed immune system only makes them harder to eliminate.

The persistent use of antibiotics and antihistamines, without judiciously removing the allergic offenders that caused the sinus infection in the first place, only results in chronic sinus infections that become resistant to therapy. The immunological reactive materials, such as free radicals, immune complexes, immunoglobulins, and peroxides, that our immune system uses to fight these chronic infections are highly toxic and must be cleared by the liver.

As one of the body's most metabolically active organs, the liver is unable to clear these toxic reactive materials without solid energy production. No surprise there. Furthermore, these toxins actually react with the mitochondria in the liver and elsewhere to decrease energy production even more.

A dangerous vicious cycle develops with age. An age-related decrease in energy production in liver cells leads to decreased liver function, which results in higher levels of these toxic immune-reactive materials circulating throughout the body. And with their negative effect on mitochondria, the escalating level of these materials causes a further decrease in energy production.

This scenario can go on for decades and can lead to a rising level of toxicity. In many cases, the treatments needed to clear these chronic sinus conditions are those which improve both energy production and liver function.

DETOXIFICATION TO THE RESCUE

The process of eliminating toxins is referred to as detoxification. Without adequate detoxification, toxins can accumulate in the tissues, and gradually, over many years, turn the body into a veritable toxic-waste dump.

Imagine how much efficiency is lost by organs trying to carry out their functions under the burden of a half-century's buildup of pollution and poison. It's easy to understand why they deteriorate at an accelerated rate. And by understanding how your body eliminates these toxins, you will be able to assist it, and prevent toxin accumulation and the inevitable decrease in energy production that comes from it.

The Lymph System

The first step in the detoxification process occurs when the cells excrete their waste products into the lymph fluid. Imagine the cells of your body aligned like a brick wall, but instead of cement, they are separated by fluid, called the lymph fluid. The lymph fluid meanders through a network of lymph ducts, and eventually dumps its cargo of wastes into the bloodstream just above the heart.

Two factors are required to assist this flow into the bloodstream. One is movement, meaning activity that moves the muscles of the arms and particularly the legs. I don't mean exercise, just the routine walking and arm movements that occur in everyday life. People who especially need to be aware of this are those with sedentary jobs where they sit for long periods of time—office workers, truck drivers, or writers, for example. If you work at such a job, be sure to get up every thirty minutes or so and walk around madly waving your arms. I'm kidding of course, but you get the idea.

The second factor is lying down. No problem there, huh? I'll bet you didn't realize that lying down was so vital to your health. Here we finally have a health concept that pretty much everyone can handle. The under-twenty age group needs about ten hours of horizontal time per twenty-four hour cycle. People over twenty need at least eight hours.

Lying down allows the lymph fluid to gravity drain. So when you sleep, the body is busy cleaning up the mess that was made during the day. Detoxification and repair are actually the primary activities of the body during sleep.

The Kidneys

After the lymph fluid is dumped into the bloodstream, the circulation carries the toxins to the kidneys and the liver. Certain toxins are selectively removed in the kidneys and dispatched to the bladder, where they are eliminated through the urine.

In order to do their jobs, the kidneys require water—pure water, and plenty of it. Not coffee, not juice, not milk, not soda—all these are liquids that may, in fact, actually impede kidney function—just water. And water is one of my secrets for better health and energy.

The Liver and Intestines

The toxins that aren't eliminated by the kidneys are processed in the liver and channeled out into the intestinal tract. Here, dietary fiber acts like a sponge and absorbs the toxins, escorting them out of the body through the feces.

This is why fiber is so important. Fiber, I should point out, is the roughage in vegetables, fruits, and whole grains. Your body doesn't absorb fiber. Instead, this material acts as a broom, keeping the intestines clean. Fiber absorbs the waste products removed by the liver, and carries them out in the stool.

People who eat diets high in processed, refined carbohydrates, such as white bread and pasta, often don't have adequate fiber. Among other harmful effects, they run the risk of having toxins reabsorbed back into the body, which just makes the liver have to work harder.

Fiber also enhances regular bowel movements and helps prevent constipation. Chronic constipation is a major cause of toxin accumulation in the tissues.

WHY YOUR LIVER IS THE MOST IMPORTANT ORGAN IN THE BODY

The body is a dynamic, interacting organism. It is affected by even the slightest alterations in the environment, as well as by diet, emotion, and thought. These influences are continually changing, of course, and the changes can easily throw the body out of balance. Not to worry however. The body has an almost miraculous ability to diagnose and correct these imbalances as they occur.

This ability is handled by the body's homeostatic regulation systems. And nothing is more important to a healthy body than the optimal functioning of these systems, which are controlled by interactions between the brain and the liver.

These two organs, the brain and the liver, are not only designed to correct homeostatic disturbances, but in fact actually require the disturbances. That's right, in order for your body to be fully healthy, it needs to be constantly challenged.

Most people would think the most important organ in this activity is the brain. And it's true that the brain has the most direct incoming and outgoing connection with all the cells and organs in the body. But it's not the most important simply because it is, for the most part, invulnerable.

The brain sits in its ivory tower like a general, separated and protected from most toxins and infections by what is known as the blood-brain barrier. This barrier allows only a very select group of molecules to come into actual contact with the brain.

Contrast this with the liver. *Unlike the brain, the liver is on the front line, where all toxins are directed.* From bacteria to viruses and pesticides, every toxin in the body must be cleared by the liver. Not only that, but it is also responsible for processing every nutrient you eat. Not a single molecule you ingest, no matter whether it's a vitamin, a mineral, fat, protein, or carbohydrate, can be used by the cells of the body until it is first processed by the liver.

Additionally, the liver regulates the balance of all the protein, fat, and carbohydrate in the blood. In combination with the spleen and intestines, the liver is the center of regulation and maintenance for the immune system. And it also regulates the balance of the entire hormonal system.

Nothing that occurs in the body is not in some major way regulated by the liver.

In contrast with the brain, moreover, the liver is not separated by a protective wall. It is right smack in the middle of all the dirty action. It is, therefore, a vulnerable organ and needs all the help and care it can get.

The fact that it is so vital to the maintenance of homeostasis, while at the same time so vulnerable to damage and dysfunction, is why I regard it as the most important organ in the body.

Let me put it another way. If you want to be healthy, do everything you can to help and protect your liver. Going forward in this book, you will see that a huge part of my program involves therapies and lifestyle habits geared to helping the liver. I have often thought it's not accidental that the word liver starts with the word *live.*

Just to review, the following basic ingredients prevent the accumulation of toxins, increase energy production, and, hence, slow down the aging process: water, fiber, sleep, movement, exercise, and nutrients that assist the liver and intestines. Along with these, it is important to try and limit exposure to toxic conditions and substances that can interfere with the elimination process by adding to the overall toxic burden. These substances include cigarette smoke, inhaled or ingested environmental chemicals, silver dental fillings, and unnecessary pharmaceutical drugs.

7

Bio-Energy Testing:
Breakthrough Technology That Tells if You Have an Energy Crisis

OK, so you have decided you want to optimize your energy production and extend the length and quality of your life. Now what? Before you can effectively start increasing your E.Q., (energy quotient) the first step is to learn exactly how good (or bad) it is, and where any potential problems may lie.

Additionally, once you get started on your re-energizing program, you will want to be able to test how effective it is and make sure it is effective enough for your genetics. Why wait until something goes wrong to learn that what you had been doing was missing a few crucial steps?

The most reliable way to determine your needs and test how well your wellness program is working for you is through Bio-Energy Testing, a unique metabolic and physiological assessment that can measure your E.Q. and much more. Thanks to Bio-Energy Testing, I can now measure every aspect of my patients' energy production easily, accurately, safely, and non-invasively. Furthermore, this technology has enabled me to discover and verify the efficacy of all the secrets presented in this book.

Each one of the secrets has been found to improve both E.Q. and Biological Age. That literally means slowing down and even reversing the aging process. I don't know this because I read about it somewhere, or because it sounds like a really good theory. I know the secrets work because I have proved it using Bio-Energy Testing with hundreds of my patients.

You may be wondering what Biological Age means. Well, your chronological age simply refers to how many years you have been alive. Your Biological Age, on the other hand, refers to how old you are from a functional standpoint. A person whose body is functioning with the efficiency typical of an older person will have a Biological Age *older* than his or her chronological age. Alternatively, a person whose body is functioning with the efficiency typical of a younger person will have a Biological Age younger than his or her chronological age.

Different anti-aging specialists have used various combinations of measurements to determine Biological Age. Such measurements include blood pressure, cholesterol levels, hearing tests, lung-function studies, vision tests, and other physiological measurements. The problem is that all these methods have flaws that limit their usefulness. The most common flaw is that the measurement being used is not consistent in everyone. Take blood-pressure measurements, for example. Although blood pressure typically elevates with age, some very young people have high blood pressure, whereas some very old people don't.

This same age-related inconsistency is seen in every measurement used to determine Biological Age—except E.Q. A decrease in E.Q. is observed in 100 percent of people as they get older. There are no exceptions.

Therefore, the research clearly shows that the most consistent and accurate way to determine Biological Age is by measuring the E.Q. For example, a seventy-five-year-old woman who has the E.Q. of a forty-five-year-old woman has a Biological Age of forty-five. And in every case I have seen over the years, she will function every bit as well as a typical forty-five-year-old woman.

Similarly, a forty-five-year-old woman with an E.Q. of a seventy-five-year-old, has a Biological Age of seventy-five, and very often will experience symptoms and other functional limitations characteristic of that older age group.

In the world of anti-aging medicine, chronological age is unimportant. It's your Biological Age that's important. That's what indicates how healthy you are, how well you feel and function, and how long you will likely live.

PRELIMINARIES TO BIO-ENERGY TESTING

Here are some insights and tips you should have prior to testing.

Older people, or anyone with heart disease, should be cleared by a physician before undertaking the exercise portion of the test. Healthy people, particularly those already exercising, can take the test without reservation.

The test is usually performed in the morning before 11 AM. You should not eat or drink anything other than water. Be extremely lazy before the

BIO-ENERGY TESTING

Bio-Energy Testing involves the use of a mouthpiece coupled with a computerized analyzer. The mouthpiece is able to measure how much oxygen the body is using and how much carbon dioxide the body is producing at any given time. These measurments are be taken at rest and also while the subject is exercising on a special computerized bicycle called an ergometer.

Additional measurements are determined using digital blood-pressure readings, body-composition measurements, and heart-rate readings.

To obtain the name of a healthcare practitioner in your area trained in the use of Bio-Energy Testing, please go to www.bioenergytesting.com.

The cost for Bio-Energy Testing will vary depending on where you have it performed, but it typically costs approximately $200. If you have a Bio-Energy test, it will be the best money you ever spend on yourself. When the test is performed by a physician, it is often reimbursible by insurance, although this will vary with the policies of each insurance company.

Before I discovered all the advantages of Bio-Energy Testing, I was the same as most anti-aging physicians. I just had to assume that the programs I put my patients on were actually working to slow down the aging process. Now, using Bio-Energy Testing, I can measure the E.Q. of every patient. And with this information I can verify whether or not my recommendations are effective. Quite simply, if it is raising the E.Q., the program is working, and if it isn't raising the E.Q., it isn't working.

When I evaluate a patient with Bio-Energy Testing, besides measuring that person's E.Q., I can also determine the following critical metabolic measurements.

※ The M-Factor (basic metabolism)

※ The C-Factor (carbohydrate factor)

※ The Fat Burning Factor (fat metabolism)

※ The maximum fat-burning heart rate (FBR) and the anaerobic-threshold heart rate (ATR). These determine your optimum exercise zone.

※ The Biological Age

※ The caloric intake for weight loss

※ The caloric intake for longevity

I will show you how these measurements are used to increase your energy levels, fine-tune your disease-prevention and anti-aging program, and improve your overall health.

Bio-Energy Testing lets me offer my patients the most efficient and accurate health, aging, and fitness assessment available. It can diagnose a decrease or an increase in E.Q., as well as pinpoint whether an energy problem is located in the adrenal glands, arteries, capillaries, heart, lungs, mitochondria, or thyroid. This makes Bio-Energy Testing the ultimate tool for anti-aging medicine, medical diagnostics, personal fitness training, and weight management.

WHAT BIO-ENERGY TESTING CAN TELL YOU

❑ Your adrenal function

❑ Your basal-metabolism rate

❑ Your Biological Age

❑ Your correct caloric intake

❑ Your E.Q. (energy quotient)

❑ Your fat/muscle ratio

❑ Your fitness level

❑ Your heart function

❑ Your lung function

❑ Your optimal weight

❑ Your optimum carbohydrate intake

❑ Your optimum exercise level for aerobic fitness

❑ Your optimum exercise level for fat loss

❑ Your thyroid function

❑ Your true anaerobic threshold

Who Can Benefit from this Test?

❑ Anyone, even an older person, who wants to feel and function like a much younger person

❑ Anyone interested in preventing the diseases of aging

❑ Anyone needing help with weight control

❑ Anyone wanting to maximize workout efficiency

❑ Anyone wanting to verify that the anti-aging program is working

❑ Anyone who is interested in slowing down the aging process

❑ Anyone with arthritis, diabetes, heart disease, or high cholesterol

❑ Chronically fatigued individuals

test—both physical and mental exertion should be kept to a minimum, and you should definitely not exercise.

Record your resting heart rate for several days prior to the test. This is done by wearing a heart-rate monitor to bed. Heart-rate monitors can be purchased at bicycle shops and sporting good stores, and typically cost around $50–$80. They come equipped with a strap outfitted with an electrode that goes over the heart. You read your heart rate on a little monitor that looks like a watch. Just before bedtime, attach the electrode. Place the monitor on a bedside stand so you can read it in the morning without having to sit up or reach over.

When you wake up, gently roll over and read your heart rate. If you had a restless night, or if you went to the bathroom within 30 minutes of waking, do not use the measurement.

Record your wake-up heart rate in this manner for several mornings. The readings should be very similar to each other. For most people, the readings will be between 55 and 70 beats per minute. People in better condition will have lower readings. Some athletes may have a resting heart rate of less than 40.

Average out your readings when you go for your Bio-Energy Test.

BASAL TESTING—THE FIRST TEST

After you arrive at the testing center, the technician will record your age, sex, height, and weight. He or she will also determine your body composition (your body's percentages of fat and muscle) using an electronic device called a bio-impedance analyzer. Your blood pressure will be taken lying down, and then again immediately after you stand up. All these measurements will be entered into the computer.

After the technician applies a heart-rate-monitor strap to your chest, you will be placed in a very comfortable reclining chair. You should be relaxed, mentally and physically, and not be concerned about the outcome of the test. Failure to adequately relax can influence the basal measurements.

Within a few minutes of settling down in the chair, the technician places the mouthpiece in your mouth, and a nose clip over your nose. The nose clip is to insure that all the air you are breathing in and out is completely recorded by the mouthpiece. There is no discomfort, so relaxing shouldn't be a problem. As you just lay back and relax, the analyzer determines how much oxygen your body is taking in, and how much carbon dioxide it is putting out.

EXERCISE TESTING

After this initial resting measurement, the fun really begins. You are placed on an ergometer, a fancy name for an exercise bicycle that uses a computer to measure how hard you are working. The seat of the cycle is adjusted so your leg is straight when the heel of your foot is on the pedal in the most extended position.

The technician again gives you the measuring mouthpiece to place in your mouth. Now you will begin to cycle. For the first several minutes, very little effort will be required of you. Then the work load on the ergomater will gradually increase, so you will have to work harder to turn the pedals. As the level of exertion increases, your heart rate will also increase. The test continues until the technician notifies you that you have entered into anaerobic energy production. At this point the test is concluded.

If you are a person who exercises regularly and is in good shape, then you will find that the exercise testing will work you pretty hard. If you are not in good shape, you will find that the exercise testing seems easy. Why? Because someone in good shape is going to be able to work much harder before becoming anaerobic than someone who is not fit.

OXYGEN CONSUMED = LIFE

Oxygen is an extremely high-energy molecule. All animals, including humans, convert oxygen, nature's highest energy molecule, to water, nature's lowest energy molecule. In this process, energy is released. *It is this precious energy that powers every aspect of your life.*

This process also generates carbon dioxide as a waste product. The amount of carbon dioxide produced is in direct proportion to the amount of energy being generated from fat, as opposed to the amount being generated from glucose.

Fortunately, all the oxygen enters the body through the lungs, and all the carbon dioxide is eliminated from the lungs. Thus, the energy-conversion process can be gauged by measuring how much oxygen and carbon dioxide are coming in and going out with each breath you take. That's precisely what the Bio-Energy Testing analyzer does.

The total amount of oxygen taken in is used to determine the total amount of energy being produced. The ratio of oxygen going in to carbon dioxide coming out is used to determine whether your body is producing energy from fat or glucose.

HOW THE BIO-ENERGY-TESTING ANALYZER KNOWS

Imagine a salesperson trying to convince a prospective buyer to buy a thermos.

"If you put something cold into it," he says, "it will stay cold. If you put in something hot, it will stay hot."

The man buys the thermos and then comes back a few weeks later.

"There's no problem at all with the thermos," he says happily. "It works great. It keeps hot things hot and cold things cold, but what I don't understand is how does it *know?*"

In order for you to understand how the Bio-Energy-Testing analyzer *knows,* take a short tour through some of the measurements used in Bio-Energy Testing, and see how they relate to the process of energy production in the body. This information can get incredibly complex, but I've attempted to keep it as simple as possible.

THE MAN BEHIND THE CURTAIN

The Bio-Energy-Testing analyzer measures the real-time breath-by-breath intake of oxygen and the production of carbon dioxide. The computer then records all the readings.

Due to the effects of coughing, sighing, and other forms of irregular breathing, there are often a few artifacts in the recorded readings that do not accurately reflect true oxygen and carbon dioxide levels. The computer program identifies these artifacts and eliminates them. It then takes the remaining readings, averages them, and uses them to make its calculations.

CALCULATING ENERGY

The oxygen that goes into the human body is primarily consumed in the mitochondria of the cells to produce energy. A small percentage of it gets used by an activated immune system when it is fighting an infection, and it can also be used by detoxification systems in the liver. But as long as the person is not actively fighting an infection, and as long as there is no acute or immediate toxicity, it can be safely assumed that all oxygen consumed is being used in the mitochondria to produce energy.

When the mitochondria produce energy, about 60 percent of it gets released as heat. The remaining 40 percent gets harnessed in the form of a molecule called adenosine triphosphate (ATP). It is ATP that every one of your cells uses to carry on its various functions. Put another way, the amount of energy your body has to perform all its functions is directly dependent on how much ATP it can produce. So when I say that Bio-Energy Testing is measuring your body's ability to produce energy, I mean that it is measuring your body's ability to produce ATP. This is how *it knows.*

The following equations show how oxygen is used in the mitochondria to produce ATP from fat:

Fat + 23 molecules of oxygen ⟶
16 molecules of carbon dioxide + 130 molecules of ATP

This equation shows that when only fat is being metabolized by oxygen to produce ATP, there is a ratio of 5.6 (130/23) molecules of ATP produced per 1 molecule of oxygen consumed. Thus, by measuring how much oxygen is consumed, the amount of ATP being produced from fat can be easily determined by multiplying this amount by 5.6.

When energy is produced from oxygen and carbohydrates (glucose), the following equations apply:

Glucose + 6 molecules of oxygen ⟶
6 molecules of carbon dioxide + 36 molecules of ATP

When glucose (the basic sugar that all carbohydrates are broken down into) is metabolized by oxygen to produce ATP, there is a ratio of six (36/6) molecules of ATP being produced per 1 molecule of oxygen being consumed. Again, simply measure oxygen consumption and you can quickly determine ATP production by multiplying this amount by 6. Note also that glucose results in 7 percent more ATP production per molecule of oxygen than fat. This is why glucose metabolism is said to be a slightly more efficient form of energy production than fat metabolism, and why the body prefers to burn glucose insttead of fat as exercise intensity increases.

Fat or Glucose?

The only problem with this particular scenario is that during the Bio-

Energy Testing procedure, the body is producing ATP from both fat and glucose. Therefore, in order to determine total ATP production with accuracy, it is necessary to know at all times what percentage of the oxygen being consumed is metabolizing glucose and what percentage is metabolizing fat.

Fortunately, the above equations can also be used to solve this problem. Notice that it is possible to determine how much fat or glucose is being metabolized by measuring the amount of carbon dioxide being simultaneously produced.

For example, when glucose is being metabolized, there is a one-to-one ratio (6:6) of carbon dioxide produced to oxygen consumed. Since the Bio-Energy Testing analyzer measures carbon-dioxide production as well as oxygen consumption, it can be determined that oxygen is metabolizing glucose exclusively when the ratio of carbon dioxide to oxygen is 1.0.

When fat is being metabolized, there is a ratio of .7 (16:23) molecules of carbon dioxide produced for every 1 molecule of oxygen being consumed. Thus, it can be determined that oxygen is metabolizing fat exclusively when the ratio of carbon dioxide to oxygen is .7.

For the mathematicians in the crowd, it is important to note that this relationship of carbon dioxide produced to oxygen consumed from fat and glucose is linear. That means it is possible to know exactly how much fat or glucose is being metabolized at all times simply by measuring the ratio of carbon dioxide to oxygen.

By constantly measuring both total oxygen being consumed and the ratio of oxygen consumed to carbon dioxide produced, the Bio-Energy-Testing analyzer is able to accurately determine two things. One, how much ATP is being produced. And two, the percentage of the ATP being produced from fat and from glucose. This may not sound like much information, but it can be used to calculate your entire energy-producing capability.

Bio-Energy Testing at a Glance

Using the information provided by the analyzer during both rest and exertion, the Bio-Energy-Testing computer program then calculates the following.

1. How much total ATP your body produces at rest.

2. How much ATP is produced just from fat at rest.

3. The maximum ATP you can produce aerobically.

4. The maximum ATP you can produce from fat.

5. The maximum amount of aerobic work your body can perform.

These calculations are then compared to what would be predicted for each individual, using standard ATP-prediction databases. The results are used to determine your M-Factor, your C-Factor, your Fat Burning Factor, your FBR (fat-burning heart rate), your ATR (anerobic-threshold heart rate), your Fitness factor, and of course, your E.Q. and your Biological Age.

Two additional factors need to be addressed regarding these calculations. They both have to do with how the determinations of predicted ATP production are calculated.

Healthy—Not Healthy for Your Age

The first factor to be addressed is age. Keep the goal in mind. From the anti-aging perspective, what you want to do is maintain youthful levels of ATP production even as you get older—you want to be healthy, not healthy for your age. Therefore, it does not make sense for older people to compare their ATP production to what is typical for their age bracket. And it isn't done in the program.

There is general agreement in the anti-aging, exercise physiology, and longevity literature, that for all practical purposes, the effects of aging do not begin to become measurable until after the age of forty. Therefore, when looking to maintain youthful levels, a reasonable benchmark for ATP production would be those levels that are typical of a forty-year-old. So, for anyone over the age of forty, all their ATP-production measurements are compared to a database with a default age of forty.

Take the case of a sixty-two-year-old woman. Her Bio-Energy-Testing results will not be comparing her to what would be considered normal and expected for the average sixty-two-year-old. Instead, the computer will compare her readings to those of the average forty-year-old woman with the same weight, and height. In other words, the goal of an anti-aging program is not to be healthy for your age. The real goal of anti-aging therapy is to be healthy for *any* age.

Since those under forty are too young to have experienced the effects of the aging process, they are compared to their own age group.

Correcting for Fat

The second factor that has to be taken into consideration for the calculation of predicted ATP production is percentage of body fat.

All of the formulas used to predict ATP production use weight as part of the input to the equation. This makes a lot of sense because it stands to reason that the more someone weighs, the bigger they are, and the more ATP they should be expected to produce. This is true for every tissue but fat. Because fat is metabolically inert tissue, it makes very little ATP. In this case, using the predictive formulas as they are classically used would result in unreasonably higher predicted levels of ATP production in anyone who has an excess of body fat. This would cause them to have a falsely elevated expectation for ATP production because of their excessive body fat. A man who weighs 200 pounds, 75 pounds of which is fat, should not be compared to a man who weights 200 pounds but only has 30 pounds of fat. The second man will obviously produce more ATP simply because he has more metabolically active tissue.

To account for this potential inaccuracy, the weight used in determining predicted ATP production is corrected. The weight of overweight men is lowered to a weight based upon an ideal body fat of 18 percent. The weight of overweight women is lowered to an ideal body fat of 22 percent.

YOUR M-FACTOR (METABOLIC FACTOR)— HOW MUCH ATP YOUR BODY PRODUCES AT REST.

Now that the right adjustments to accurately predict ATP production have been made, take a look at what Bio-Energy Testing is going to tell about how much ATP you make. By measuring how much ATP your body produces at rest, the Bio-Energy-Testing analyzer can determine your basal metabolic rate (BMR). Your BMR reflects your overall metabolism. Those with high BMRs have high metabolic rates, and those with low BMRs have low metabolic rates.

Your BMR is especially valuable for weight control because it is used to compute how many calories your body will burn in a day. It is also a much more accurate way to diagnose low-thyroid states than blood testing.

Dietitians have used many formulas to estimate BMR, but for most people, especially those for whom it is the most important, these estimates are almost always inaccurate. Bio-Energy Testing is unique in that it precisely measures your exact BMR. Once your BMR is measured, your M-Factor can be determined.

For people younger than forty, the M-Factor is equal to the ratio of their measured BMR as determined by Bio-Energy Testing, compared to the average BMR of a healthy person the same age, weight, height, and gender.

For those over forty, the M-Factor equals the ratio of the measured BMR compared to the average BMR of a healthy forty-year-old the same weight, height, and gender. The optimal M-Factor is 100 percent. This would indicate that the person being tested is producing the entire amount of ATP that is predicted.

Since the M-Factor declines with aging, it is an excellent yardstick of your rate of aging. But it is not only an excellent way to determine how well your anti-aging program is working, it also supplies the critical information needed to establish the correct therapeutic program for optimum energy production and weight control.

A 2004 study underlines this fact. Based on their M-Factor, the researchers looked at how long individual mice lived. What they found was that the mice with the highest M-Factors lived a whopping 36-percent longer than the mice with the lowest readings—an astounding testimony to the effect of resting ATP production.

Low M-Factors aren't just a result of getting older. They also decline from disease. And they vary considerably from person to person depending on diet, genetics, fitness, and hormone levels (particularly thyroid and adrenal hormones). Nutrient deficiencies, especially the B vitamins, coenzyme Q_{10}, fatty acids, and magnesium, can also play a significant role in determining the M-Factor.

Your M-Factor can signal significant decreases in thyroid function (hypothyroidism) that often go undiagnosed. A low M-Factor is the most sensitive indicator of low-thyroid states, even when thyroid blood tests show normal values. (*See* Chapter 15, Secret Eight.)

YOUR C-FACTOR—
HOW MUCH ATP IS PRODUCED FROM FAT AT REST

As stated above, when glucose is being metabolized, there is a one-to-one ratio of carbon dioxide produced to oxygen consumed. When fat is being metabolized, the ratio is .7. Since the Bio-Energy-Testing analyzer measures carbon-dioxide production as well as oxygen consumption, the percentage of fat being metabolized can be determined by examining this ratio.

Based on my own measurements and those published, when a healthy person is resting, she/he should be able to produce at least 75 percent of his or her total ATP production from fat. I have measured some competitive athletes who made almost 90 percent of their resting ATP from fat. But this is a super-human level. Seventy-five percent is more than enough, but less than that indicates decreased fat metabolism. Since fat provides most of our overall energy, decreased fat metabolism causes major decreases in total energy production.

The reason the body can't produce 100 percent of its resting energy from fat has to do with the brain. Unlike every other organ in the body, the brain can utilize only glucose for energy. Since the brain is active even in a resting state, there is always going to be some glucose metabolism going on in the brain.

Once the percentage of resting ATP production from fat is measured by the analyzer, the computer presents it as the C-Factor. The C-Factor is formulated on a scale of 50–100 as shown below.

☀ A C-Factor of 100 indicates that 75 percent of the resting ATP is from fat. This points to optimal resting fat metabolism.

☀ A C-Factor less than 100 indicates that progressively less than 75 percent of the resting ATP is from fat. This points to impaired resting fat metabolism. For example, a C-Factor of 80 indicates that only 50 percent of the resting ATP production is from fat.

☀ A C-Factor of 50 indicates that none of the resting ATP is coming from fat, it is all coming from glucose. This points to a severe impairment of resting fat metabolism.

Why Is It Called C-Factor?

It turns out that when you are at rest, the amount of carbohydrate in your diet determines how much fat your body is burning more than any other single factor. The more carbohydrate you eat, the less fat you will burn. The reason is actually quite simple. When you feed your body carbohydrates, it will take the most energy-efficient path it can. Rather than store the carbohydrates for later use and in the meanwhile rely on fat metabolism, it will just take the easy way out and burn the carbohydrates for energy.

The more carbohydrate you eat, the less fat your body will need to burn. If you eat enough carbohydrate, your body will not need to burn any fat at all. This effect of dietary carbohydrate on fat metabolism is the most common single cause of decreased energy production that I see.

This suppressive effect of carbohydrate on fat burning is quite individual. There are some people who can have a relatively high intake of carbohydrates and yet still maintain an optimal C-Factor. Most people, however, need to maintain a very modest intake of carbohydrates in order to avoid suppressing fat metabolism.

Let me offer a very graphic case example to make my point.

A forty-two-year-old movie actor came to my clinic to have his energy production analyzed with Bio-Energy Testing. He was an avid exerciser, and took an array of supplements as part of an anti-aging/preventive medicine program. He had no complaints, and his physical and routine laboratory examinations were almost completely normal. The only problem he had was a modest elevation of a blood fat called triglyceride. When I first saw him, I thought this young man looked like the epitome of health. Looks can be deceiving however, especially in health because, when tested, this man had an E.Q. of only 60%. That placed him in the category of a severe energy deficit.

Additionally, his C-Factor was 50. This meant his resting energy production from fat was zero. Essentially, he had no fat metabolism. He was spending his days living strictly off his carbohydrate stores.

I have learned not to be too surprised by such findings, and I immediately asked him about his diet. He then confessed that every day for the previous two months he had been consuming two milk shakes blended with cookies at a popular fast food restaurant.

I asked him to continue everything he was currently doing except drinking the milk shakes. I also asked him to avoid all other carbohydrates, including fruit, grains, legumes, sugars, and tubers.

He repeated his Bio-Energy Testing in three weeks and was much happier the second time around. In only three weeks his E.Q. had more than tripled. It had increased to 130 of percent that of the average man two years younger. From energetic rags to riches in only three weeks simply by dramatically decreasing dietary carbohydrate.

Not surprisingly, this second test revealed that his C-Factor was now maximal at 101. Cases such as this form the majority of what I see on a daily basis in my clinic. So if you haven't already figured it out by now, that's why resting fat metabolism is presented as C-Factor. The C stands for carbohydrate.

❊ A C-Factor equal to 100 indicates you are eating an optimal amount of carbohydrate for your genetics and lifestyle.

❊ A C-Factor less than 100 indicates that for your genetics and lifestyle your intake of carbohydrates is excessive, and is impairing your fat metabolism.

❊ A C-Factor of 50 indicates that your intake of carbohydrates is so excessive, it is completely suppressing all fat metabolism.

It is important to note here that resting fat metabolism can be impaired by factors other than carbohydrates. Every now and then I see a person who is on a very low carbohydrate diet, but who still has a low C-Factor. This can happen because resting fat metabolism is also influenced by other factors.

Deficiencies of the adrenal hormones cortisol and DHEA, the anabolic hormones HGH, progesterone, and testosterone, and the thyroid hormones T_4 and T_3 also play a significant role. Other routinely encountered factors include deficiencies of amino acids, B vitamins, chromium, co-enzyme Q_{10}, essential fats, L-carnitine, lipoic acid, and magnesium. All these nutrients are especially likely to be deficient in people who eat excessive amounts of carbohydrates. In addition, excessive dietary intake of trans-fatty acids, insulin resistance, and sleep deprivation are also factors affecting resting fat metabolism. However, in a resting state the demand for ATP is pretty minimal, so these factors usually have only a small effect on the C-Factor score compared to the carbohydrate effect.

If your C-Factor is low, particularly if it is less than 90, you are eating too many carbohydrates for optimal energy production. Sometimes the amount of dietary carbohydrate that will suppress fat metabolism is quite small. In fact, after observing the C-Factors of hundreds of my patients, I can report there are a great many people out there who seem to be genetically programmed so that, in order to optimally burn fat, they must eat almost no carbohydrate at all.

WHY IS THE C-FACTOR IMPORTANT?

The C-Factor is important because it specifically looks at resting fat metabolism, how well you are burning fat to make energy when you are in a resting state. (A resting state is when you are not exerting.)

A hundred years ago, before cars, central heating, washing machines, and other conveniences people now take for granted, the everyday lifestyle involved much more exertion. In fact, people probably spent most of their waking hours in acitivities that involved exertion.

But today, most people are like me. I drive to work. My work consists of sitting down all day and walking from one room to another. When I get home, I exercise for thirty minutes, then I rest from my hard day of mental activity. And finally, I go to sleep for eight hours, and start all over again.

On the weekends, I might work in the garden, ride my horse, sail my boat, or set out on a bike ride. The point I am making is, except for my daily thirty minutes of exercise, I am in a resting state for twenty-three and a half hours every day. So, for me, and for every one of you who has a similar contemporary lifestyle, resting fat metabolism is critically important—because that's the state people are in 98 percent of the time.

The three most important considerations for your overall health are your resting overall metabolism (M-Factor), your resting fat metabolism (C-Factor), and your mitochondrial function (E.Q.). Two out of these three measurements are resting measurements. And the reason they are so important is because 98 percent of the time the majority of people are in a resting state.

The fact that you can burn fat well while exercising is relatively unimportant. What you do in your resting state is really what it is all about. And that's why your C-Factor measurement is so critical to your health.

FAT BURNING FACTOR—
MAXIMAL ATP PRODUCTION FROM FAT

Once the resting energy-production readings have been determined, Bio-Energy Testing then determines how well your mitochondria are functioning. It does this by examining how well you can make ATP while exercising. This part of the test uses a specialized stationary bicycle called an ergometer.

The resistance on the ergometer refers to how hard it is to turn the pedals. It is controlled by a computer. The higher the resistance is set, the more you will have to work to turn the pedals. The more fit you are, the harder the resistance will be set. The more out of shape you are, the easier the resistance. That way, everyone can be evaluated according to their own particular level of fitness. Once you start exercising on the ergometer, the computer will steadily increase the resistance every fifteen seconds. This will cause you to steadily work harder and harder.

As your exertion increases, your rising energy demands will cause your body to metabolize increasing amounts of fat into ATP. And so, as the resistance becomes harder and harder, your body will be burning more and more fat.

This increase in fat burning can only go on for a limited amount of time, however, because fat metabolism is not as fast and energy-efficient as glucose metabolism. Therefore, as the resistance becomes harder and your energy demands continue to increase, your body will start to shift from burning fat to burning glucose.

At some point during the test you will reach a level of exertion where you are burning the maximum amount of fat your body is able to metabolize. As you continue to exercise beyond this point and your need for ATP steadily increases, you will be metabolizing progressively more glucose and less fat. This point of maximum fat burning can be determined by the Bio-Energy-Testing analyzer. It is used to determine your Fat-Burning factor.

As exercise intensity continues to increase, you will eventually get to a point where you are metabolizing no fat at all. At this second point, all ATP production will come entirely from glucose. Called the anaerobic threshold, this marks the point where you have reached your maximal aerobic ATP production.

Your Fat-Burning factor refers to the maximal amount of ATP you can produce from fat. Like the other Bio-Energy-Testing factors, it is a percentage calculation, which compares your measurement to one expected from a healthy person your sex, height, and weight. Based on my own measurements and those published, a healthy person should be able to produce at least 60 percent of her or his maximal aerobic ATP production from fat. Less than that indicates impaired fat metabolism.

The computer determines your Fat-Burning factor and presents it in the following way.

☀ A Fat-Burning factor equal to 100 indicates your body is able to produce at least 60 percent of your maximal aerobic ATP production from fat. This points to optimal fat metabolism.

☀ A Fat-Burning factor less than 100 indicates you are producing less than 60 percent of your maximal aerobic ATP production from fat. This points to less than optimal fat metabolism.

☀ A Fat-Burning factor less than 70 indicates you are producing less than 30 percent of your maximal aerobic ATP production from fat. This points to a severe impairment of fat metabolism.

I want you to be healthy, not just healthy for your age. Therefore, for anyone younger than forty, the Fat-Burning factor compares them to healthy people the same age, weight, height, and gender. But for those over forty, the Fat-Burning factor compares them to healthy people the same weight, height, and gender who are forty-years-old.

THE DIFFERENCE BETWEEN C-FACTOR AND FAT-BURNING FACTOR

The difference between C-Factor and Fat-Burning factor is as follows. The C-Factor is a measurement of resting fat metabolism. Resting fat metabolism is almost always a function of carbohydrate intake. So if your C-Factor is decreased, you can bet that you are eating too many carbohydrates.

The Fat-Burning factor is not as influenced by carbohydrate intake as the C-Factor. It is more affected by other determinants of fat metabolism. These other determinants include dietary deficiencies of essential fats, excessive dietary intake of trans-fatty acids, insulin resistance, and sleep deprivation. They also include deficiencies of B vitamins, chromium, coenzyme Q_{10}, L-carnitine, hormones, lipoic acid, magnesium, and toxicity.

Additionally, the C-Factor and Fat-Burning-factor measurements are very important for people who find it hard to maintain a healthy weight. They often have a low C-Factor along with a low Fat-Burning factor. Functionally speaking, that means the majority of their daily energy needs are being met by carbohydrate metabolism. No wonder they can't lose weight. *They can't burn fat.*

FAT—YOUR PRIMARY ENERGY SOURCE

Fat has received an enormous amount of negative press over the years. Yet, fat is absolutely central to energy production. Many nutritionists still profess that carbohydrate is the body's primary energy source. But they are wrong.

My use of Bio-Energy Testing has taught me an amazing fact: A decline in fat metabolism is more responsible for the effects of aging and degenerative disease than any other single factor. This is because fat is the body's ideal energy raw material. Nature designed it that way.

Here's why. Every time you eat, the energy from the meal is stored as fat. If you eat fat, it gets stored as fat. And if you eat carbohydrate, it get stored as fat. In terms of increasing your fat stores, it makes no difference what you eat. Both carbohydrates and fats get stored as fat. And there's a very good reason for this. The human body has evolved over many thousands of years. Genetic testing has revealed there is essentially no difference at all between its metabolism today and the metabolism that existed in ancient ancestors.

But unlike now, our ancestors were never quite sure of their next meal. They could easily go days to weeks before eating again. They needed to have a way of storing up energy for those long gaps between suppers. And that's where fat comes in. It can store more than twice as much energy as carbohydrates. Furthermore, the body has evolved the capability of storing huge amounts of fat, whereas it can only store a tiny amount of carbohydrates. Add these two facts up. If carbohydrates are the main energy provider for cells, then Mother Nature must be pretty stupid.

I discovered the amazing value of fat quite by accident. It happened as I was analyzing the Bio-Energy-Testing results of several hundred of people. As I studied the data, I gradually became aware of a certain pattern. The younger, healthier, and more athletic a person was, the more efficiently he or she burned fat. However, the older or sicker people were, the less energy they produced from fat metabolism, and the more they began to obtain their energy needs from carbohydrates.

The average healthy twenty-two-year-old would obtain close to 80 percent of daily energy needs from fat. But by the time this individual reaches fifty-five-years-old, she or he would be lucky to be producing half the needed energy from fat. As people aged or developed illnesses, I saw this consistent shift from fat metabolism to carbohydrate metabolism over and over again.

A decrease in energy production from fat results in a corresponding decrease in total energy production. This is because, outside of an occasional brief period of exertion, fat is the major source of energy in the healthy body.

The fact that fat metabolism plays the key role in energy production is emphasized in many research papers. In a 2002 paper, researchers were able to restore youthful levels of fat metabolism to a group of old rats. When they did this, they were able to restore the aging rats' energy production to that typical of younger rats, "thus delaying mitochondrial decay and aging." They proved that better fat metabolism = better energy production.

ARE YOU BURNING FAT EFFICIENTLY?

Is it any wonder obesity is now considered epidemic in the United States? We have these Paleolithic metabolisms that are designed to go long times without eating. But instead of going without food, three squares a day has become the reality. We truly have caveman bodies living in a supermarket world.

The constant eating, combined with high-carbohydrate and low-fat intake, has just about completely shut down the nation's fat metabolism. But the evolutionary process of storing meals as fat has not changed. We can store the fat, but we can't burn it. The result? The perfect recipe for weight gain.

When the body cannot burn fat efficiently, it will pile up the fat stores. But that's not all. Because it is storing up all this energy instead of burning it, it will have dramatically low levels of energy production. And the resulting low energy only serves to speed the aging process at an ever-increasing rate.

Aging, gaining weight, low energy, and disease all go hand in hand. They're just different sides of the same problem—an inability to burn or metabolize fat. There are two proofs of this. One is the fact that an increase in body fat is one of the most consistent hallmarks of the aging process. The other is that the risk for developing every disease from cancer to diabetes is increased in those who are fat.

And, despite what you may hear from many so-called experts in the diet industry, excessive carbohydrate consumption—and not fat—is the major dietary cause of weight gain. It also is the leading cause of diabetes and high cholesterol. In my practice, only about one in twenty patients puts on weight by eating too much fat.

It seems like a reasonable enough assumption that eating fat causes fat gain, but the science doesn't support it for the great majority of people.

Perhaps the most useful measurements of Bio-Energy Testing are the C-Factor and the Fat-Burning factor. These determine how well you metabolize fat. And how well you burn fat is critical to your health because it accounts for the majority of your overall energy production.

DETERMINING YOUR E.Q.

Your E.Q., or energy quotient, is a measurement of your maximal aerobic-energy production. It tells you how well your body is able to produce energy from oxygen. If your E.Q. is high, then you are highly efficient at producing energy from oxygen. If it is low, the opposite is the case.

A high E.Q. means you are in an optimum state of health. A low E.Q. means your health is in jeopardy. You are aging faster than you should, as well as increasing your risk for every disease, from cancer to arthritis.

During the exercise part of Bio-Energy Testing, your exertion level is steadily increased until you get to your anaerobic threshold. This is your point of maximal aerobic-energy production. At this point, your body is producing ATP from oxygen as efficiently as it can.

The Bio-Energy-Testing analyzer measures how much ATP you are producing at this point. Then the computer program compares your ATP production to that expected for the average healthy person. Just as with the other measurements, for anyone younger than forty, the computer compares them to healthy persons their age, weight, height, and gender. But for those over forty, it compares them to forty-year-old healthy people the same weight, height, and gender.

The computer determines your E.Q.and presents the results in this way.

☀ An E.Q. greater than 100 indicates your body is able to produce ATP from oxygen at a very healthy level. This points to optimal health.

☀ An E.Q. less than 100 indicates your body is not able to produce adequate levels of ATP from oxygen. This points to less than optimal health, accelerated aging, and increased risk of disease.

✳ An E.Q. less than 66 indicates your body is only able to produce less than 66 percent of the amount of ATP it needs to be healthy. This points to a severe impairment of ATP production. It means your mitochondria are in a true state of emergency. Your body is aging much too rapidly, and is on the fast track towards disease.

YOUR E.Q. AT WORK

Take a look at what this means in principle. It's time to brag now.

Suppose you are like me, a sixty-year-old man who does all kinds of things to be healthy. You have a special diet you stick to. You have a regular exercise program. You work on not getting overly stressed. You take nutritional supplements and, just as I do, you also take supplementary hormones to boost your sagging levels.

Then suppose you have your energy-production efficency determined using Bio-Energy Testing. Your E.Q. turns out to be 130 (as mine was recently). What does this mean? Well, it's really good news.

An E.Q. of 130 means your body is producing energy 30 percent more efficiently than a man twenty years younger. It means you are aging at a snail's pace. It also means your risk of developing disease is at an all-time low. It is basically the same risk that the average thirty-year-old has. What risk is that? Essentially no risk at all.

But there's even more good news. Such a wonderful E.Q. reading confirms in your mind that all the measures you are taking to slow aging down and stay healthy are working for your particular genetics. In other words, you are not wasting your time, energy, and money on a program that will not deliver.

But what if you don't come out with an E.Q. as good as mine? What if, like many of my patients, your E.Q. is less than 100 the first time I measure it? What does that mean?

Well, first of all, it is good news. It tells you in no uncertain terms that your health program is not working with your particular genetics. So, rather than continuing an ineffective regimen, you and your healthcare practitioner can use the information from your Bio-Energy Testing to come up with a program that will work.

There is no one health program that will work for everyone—this is just common sense. For some people, a vegetarian diet is just what they need. For others, such a diet spells disaster. The same is true for supplements, hormones, exercise programs, etc. Bio-Energy Testing is essential to know if all those things you do to stay healthy are in fact really working.

THE FERRARI AND THE CLUNKER

I'll turn to the automotive world for a moment and put you behind the wheel of a brand new Ferrari to illustrate my point.

The tank is filled with the highest octane gasoline available to accommodate the Ferrari's high-performance engine. The fuel pump and the carburetor are delivering the gas to the cylinders. The spark plugs are new. The battery has plenty of juice.

This is analogous to you having good lungs, a good heart, and good circulation. Everything is set for a great ride.

But what if the engine is out of tune? That new Ferrari will run no better than an old clunker. In fact, a well-tuned old clunker will most surely outperform a poorly tuned new Ferrari.

When your body is highly tuned, your E.Q. will be 100 or higher.

Nothing is more tied to mental and physical functioning and disease prevention than optimum energy production as manifested by an optimum E.Q.

YOUR FBR—FAT-BURNING HEART RATE

Are you keeping up so far? Just remember that your M-Factor directly correlates with aging, health, and weight management. It can signal significant decreases in thyroid function (hypothyroidism) that might otherwise go undiagnosed.

Your C-Factor should be greater than 100. If it isn't, that means you're probably eating too many carbohydrates, and your energy production from fat is being suppressed as a result.

Your Fat-Burning factor should be greater than 100. If it's not, then you are not burning fat efficiently. This could happen from eating too many carbohydrates, but it could also indicate various nutritional or hormonal deficiencies.

Your E.Q. should be greater than 100. That way you can be assured your health and anti-aging program is really living up to your expectations.

Now look at how Bio-Energy Testing can help you dial in your exercise program. During the exercise part of the test, as you continue to work harder and harder, your body will burn more and more fat to meet your increased energy needs. But, there will be a point at which your body has reached its maximum level of fat burning. This is where your Fat-Burning factor is determined. I refer to the heart rate at this point as the fat-burning heart rate, or FBR.

Your FBR defines your point of recovery during your exercise period. By point of recovery, I mean the point at which your body is able to recover from the stress and strain of hard exercise. It is important for your exercise period to include a significant amount of time at your point of recovery.

Why? Because the body always responds best to a stimulus when it is repetitive and not continuous. Your brain, for example, will learn best if you alternate periods of learning with periods of mental rest. Your muscles will also respond better if you work them and then rest them, rather than continually stressing them and not allowing for a recovery period. In order to be really effective, therefore, all exercise programs must have hard, challenging periods of time alternating with periods during which the body can recover.

This is one reason why knowing your FBR is so valuable. The other has to do with exercising for fat loss. When you are exercising at your FBR, your body is burning fat as fast as it can. You are training your body to burn fat more efficiently when you are exercising at your FBR. When your exercise intensity drives your heart rate beyond your FBR, the proportion of energy produced from fat metabolism declines, and your body begins to burn carbohydrates instead. So, exercising above your FBR is actually counterproductive for fat loss.

Time and time again I see frustrated patients who are overweight in spite of the fact they are exercising harder and harder. The problem? They are exercising too hard. They are spending no time at all at their FBR, and their entire exercise period is only training their body to burn carbohydrates, not fat. No wonder it doesn't work.

A few years ago, I published an article, "Is your patient exercising too hard to be healthy?" which stressed this fact. It can be found in Appendix B and I highly recommend you read it if weight control is an issue for you. But whether you want to lose weight or not, it is always better to spend a significant part of your exercise at your FBR.

YOUR ATR—ANAEROBIC-THRESHOLD HEART RATE

As you keep on exercising harder and harder and your heart rate escalates beyond your FBR, you will eventually reach a point of exercise called your anaerobic threshold. At this point, your cells have completely maxed out their production of ATP from oxygen. I refer to your heart rate when you reach your anaerobic threshold as your ATR, or anaerobic-threshold heart rate (not to be confused with an ATM).

Exercising at your ATR forces your mitochondria to make energy as efficiently as possible. It also maximizes your circulation, stimulates your detoxification systems, and strengthens your heart and lungs more than any other point of exercise.

This is the point of exercise where you have your maximum total aerobic-training effect. So whenever you exercise, you want to be sure to spend some time at your ATR. (*See* Chapter 13, Secret Six.)

While exercising at your ATR immensely benefits your overall health, exercising *above* your ATR for any length of time is very unhealthy. Why? As soon as you go above your ATR, your body starts to produce ATP without oxygen. This kind of energy production is called anaerobic metabolism, and it is very undesirable, which is why it is so important to know your ATR.

Anaerobic energy production causes increased free-radical damage in the body. It also puts the adrenal glands into a hyper state, which ultimately leads to their exhaustion, and it creates a high tide of tissue-acid production.

One way to experience how anaerobic-energy production can feel is to just hold your breath. It will take you less than a minute of this to figure out a few things about anaerobic metabolism.

1. You will soon become energy-deprived. Anaerobic- energy production can only meet your energy demands for a very limited amount of time because the production of energy in the body from anaerobic metabolism is only a fraction (1/18) of that produced when oxygen is used.

2. Since the brain is the most sensitive organ to energy-deficiency states, it panics and eventually can't function.

3. It usually hurts because anaerobic metabolism produces a huge amount of acid, and excessive acid causes pain in the muscles.

4. You become breathless because anaerobic metabolism causes a buildup of carbon dioxide, which is what drives your breathing rate.

Now imagine someone who has a low E.Q. and can't produce ATP well from oxygen. When he exerts himself, that person's body will be forced into producing ATP anerobically much sooner than someone with a healthy E.Q. He will often experience many of the above symptoms, even at very low levels of exertion.

Over the years I have been astounded to see many people with E.Q.'s so low that they go into anaerobic metabolism simply by walking across the room. These people are commonly labeled with chronic fatigue syndrome or fibromyalgia. They often complain of all of the symptoms associated with anaerobic metabolism, including anxiety and panic states, breathlessness, mental confusion, muscle aches and pains, a profound lack of endurance, and severe fatigue. Unless the causes of their decreased E.Q. are successfully addressed, their lives are quite limited.

YOUR BIOLOGICAL AGE—
HOW OLD ARE YOU REALLY?

Alas, aerobic-energy production steadily decreases with age. And other factors, such as decreased fitness, excessive carbohydrates, illness, nutrient and hormonal deficiencies, stress, and toxicity, can compound the problem.

This decline results in a diminished function in every single cell, organ, and tissue in the body, and is behind all the symptoms and diseases of aging. Since the brain, the heart, and the liver are the largest consumers of energy in the body, these organs are the most affected. But the bad news is—no part of your body is spared.

The good news is that, even though your energy-producing efficiency may be decreased, using the guidelines provided from Bio-Energy Testing, you still have the potential to improve dramatically. Studies have clearly shown that maximizing your energy production is the best way to feel great, prevent disease, and slow down aging.

Your age only reflects how long you have been alive, and other than spending more for life insurance, or getting into the movies for less, your age turns out to be relatively unimportant. What is important is how efficiently your body is able to produce energy. That's what determines your health, your rate of aging, and your resistance to disease—*and that's what your Biological Age is all about.*

In determining your Biological Age, the computer matches your total energy dynamics with people your sex, height, and weight of various ages.

If your Biological Age is less than your chronological age, congratulations—you have just cheated Mother Nature out of the aging process. You can rest assured that all the time, energy, and money you spend to keep healthy is really doing what it's supposed to do.

If your Biological Age is greater than your chronolical age, congratulations as well because, instead of continuing a lifestyle and supplement program that isn't working, you are now armed with the right information to make the needed changes. You may be a clunker now, but you have the potential to perform like a new Ferrari. If you follow up your new program with Bio-Energy Testing, you will be able to confirm that it is effective. By determining your Biological Age, you can know how old you *really* are— no matter how many candles they stick in your birthday cake.

Now that you are familiar with the importance of these vital Bio-Energy-Testing measurements, it's time to move on and introduce you to the practical steps you can take to improve each and every reading.

PART TWO

Eight Secrets
for Improving
Your Energy

8

Secret One—
Water

Water has absolutely no nutritional value. Your body cannot produce energy from water. Nevertheless, all energy production, and indeed life itself would very quickly come to a halt without water.

You can go without eating for weeks, but you cannot go without water for more than several days. The reason: 75 percent of your body is comprised of water, and every single aspect of your biological functioning will quickly break down without enough water in your system.

A very simple home experiment can demonstrate this. Put a bit of baking soda and vitamin-C powder into a glass. What happens? Absolutely nothing! Now add a little water and watch the powerful reaction that develops. In your body the same effect is at work.

Without adequate amounts of water, every biochemical reaction, including those essential for the proper generation of energy, is compromised. Take the brain. It is an organ with highly complex biochemical reactivity. The speed at which these reactions occur is critical, your information processing and thinking activity depend on it. While most other organs in the body are made up of 75 percent water, the brain consists of 85 percent water. When it becomes even slightly dehydrated, your mental speed declines markedly, and greater levels of dehydration result in delirium and seizures.

Another critical aspect of water relates to detoxification. *Water is the only solvent the body can use to rid itself of toxins.* Some toxins are environmental and enter the body, but the majority are formed inside the body as the waste products of normal metabolic function. Without any water intake, these toxins would accumulate so rapidly that, in most cases, you would die within four or five days. With a much less-than-optimal intake you wouldn't die, but you wouldn't be able to flush the toxins out fast enough, and this would lead to toxin accumulation, decreased energy production, decreased organ function, and ultimately disease.

Yet another vital function of water is the maintenance of body temperature. Your body's ability to cool itself depends on adequate water intake. High fevers associated with acute illnesses, such as the flu, are often the result of dehydration. And if you are intolerant of hot weather, chances are you are significantly dehydrated. Think of water as the coolant you put in your car. If the level goes down too far, the engine overheats. It's the same with your body.

FEW PEOPLE DRINK ENOUGH

Despite its fundamental importance, it is amazing how few people actually drink enough water. In my clinic, I find that many of my healthy preventive-medicine patients are somewhat dehydrated. They all state that they feel great and have no symptoms, yet when I check their body's water level they are clearly deficient.

And when asked if they are thirsty, none of them ever respond positively. Although thirst is a pretty good indicator of *acute* dehydration, in chronic states of dehydration the body adjusts by retaining fluids, so thirst does not occur.

Thirst turns out to be a poor indicator of whether or not you have an adequate level of water in your body. A 1998 article in the *American Journal of Hospital Palliative Care* dramatically points this out. The researchers reported that fluid depletion, even in severely dehydrated, dying people resulted "in relatively benign symptoms," of which thirst was not a common one. The bottom line here is, just because you're not thirsty, doesn't mean you may not be dehydrated. The only way to be sure you have adequate water levels in your body is to drink plenty of water.

When the body retains fluids in a state of dehydration, it is also retaining the toxins that those fluids were supposed to eliminate. This increases the level of toxins in your tissues, and sets the stage for chronic disease and premature aging.

Fereydoon Batmanghelidj, M.D., an expert on water and author of an excellent book, *Your Body's Many Cries for Water,* points out that the body has no water-storage system to draw on in times of need. And those parts of the body most acutely affected by a water shortage are the areas without a direct blood supply, particularly cartilage in the joints. Painful joints, including those with arthritis in them, can be a result of inadequate water intake, Batmanghelidj says.

This overlooked issue was singled out in *Preventing Arthritis*, a book by Ronald M. Lawrence, M.D., Ph.D., a pain specialist. "I have indeed found that joint and pain problems are helped by water, and made worse when a patient is dehydrated or hardly drinks water at all," he says.

CURED WITH WATER

Years ago, Sarah, a seventy-two-year-old woman, made an appointment to see me and reported the following medical history. Eight months earlier she had started to experience nausea. Her appetite had gradually diminished and she had begun to lose weight. Her physician had prescribed various medications, including ulcer drugs, but nothing improved her condition. Two months went by, and Sarah began to develop a severe pain in her right hip. Her doctor knew she had arthritis damage in this hip, and concluded that the increase in pain meant it was finally time for a hip replacement.

After several weeks of continued pain, she was admitted to the hospital and had the surgery. Following the procedure, her nausea worsened to the point that she vomited almost everything she ate. She was prescribed more pain medication, and was ultimately placed on significantly high doses of strong narcotics. She was then discharged from the hospital, but returned with continued nausea, weight loss, and vomiting (no complaint about thirst).

Scans, X-rays, and blood tests failed to reveal any abnormality, but since it was obvious she was dehydrated, she was treated for fluid replacement with intravenous salt water. Miraculously, her symptoms improved, and after the third day she was allowed to return home.

Two months later, Sarah came to my clinic complaining of persistent joint pain, continued dependence on narcotic medication, and relentless nausea and vomiting. The case stumped me. I tried a homeopathic approach, but was unable to make any inroads. It was not until I recommended she drink six ounces of water every hour that the situation changed.

Within several days, she had completely turned around. The stomach symptoms disappeared. The pain went away. It turned out that Sarah's **entire** range of symptoms was due to dehydration. Had she been adequately hydrated from the beginning, she may have been able to avoid the surgery, and all the misery she experienced during those many months. Remarkably, during the entire time, Sarah never once complained of thirst.

WATER PURITY

When I talk to my patients about water, I emphasize the importance of *pure* water. Regular tap water is often contaminated by chlorine, fluoride, hard minerals, heavy metals, or pesticide residues. This means the water not only carries toxins with it into your body, but these toxins actually reduce its important solvent duties once inside.

Don't assume your water source is clean. According to a 1993 statement from the Environmental Protection Agency, 819 cities across the United States serve up unacceptably elevated levels of lead to some 30,000,000 customers. Additionally, one-fourth of all the public water systems in the United States have been found in violation of federal standards for water purity. Several epidemics of infectious diseases have been traced to contaminated public and ground water, and have led to recalls of meats and vegetables.

I have been testing water for many years, and rarely do I find any well or city water pure enough to generate optimum detoxifying effects in the body. To counter this, I recommend that my patients install a home purification unit. The key word here is *purified*. Water labeled as drinking water, mineral water, or spring water, is just not pure enough. Ideally, water should be purified using either a reverse osmosis or distillation method. My favorite is reverse osmosis because distillation units are complex, expensive, and don't remove as many potentially harmful materials.

My Recommendations to You

❋ Drink at least one-quarter to one-half your weight in ounces of water per day. If you have joint or muscle aches, try drinking the maximum for a few weeks to see if it makes a difference. For example, if you weigh 180 pounds, drink a minimum of 45 ounces daily (that's approximately six eight-ounce glasses of water.

❋ On hot days, or when exercising, twice that amount may be needed.

❋ Once your body is used to drinking this amount of water, you will begin to feel thirsty if you aren't getting enough. But as a rule, don't rely on thirst to remind you to drink water.

❋ Since your lymphatic system has been collecting toxins and dumping them into your bloodstream during the night, it's good to get into the habit of helping the kidneys by drinking sixteen to thirty-two ounces of water when you get up in the morning. This may take some getting used to, but it's worth it.

❋ Alcohol drinks, coffee, juice, sodas, and tea are not water. Nor are they substitutes for water. In fact, through their diuretic action, they can actually intensify dehydration.

9

Secret Two— Rest

Get plenty of rest. That's the age-old physician prescription for sickness. It's also an age-old prescription for staying healthy. And today, even in this time of medical marvels, it still holds true because nothing is more critical to optimal energy production than sleep.

I find that the issue of adequate rest and sleep appears to be a major challenge for my patients. I am constantly reminding them that rest is really important—not getting enough of it can be a major barrier to all their health and anti-aging goals. Yet, often it doesn't really sink in. Perhaps it's just too simple a concept.

And the attitude of catching up on lost sleep "when I have the time" just doesn't cut it. Without adequate sleep, your metabolic rate and your E.Q. will decrease. Sleep-deprivation shortens your life and increases the likelihood of a variety of diseases including cancer, diabetes, and obesity.

My observation over the years has been that those people who sleep the best also feel the best. They are the healthiest ones.

According to a 1997 article in the *New York Times Magazine*, many sleep researchers believe that sleep deprivation is reaching "crisis proportions." This is not just a problem for serious insomniacs, but for the populace at large, the article said, and added, "People don't merely believe they're sleeping less, they are *in fact* sleeping less—perhaps as much as one and a half hours less each night than humans did at the beginning of the century—often because they choose to do so."

In an October 2000 report published in the British journal *Occupational and Environmental Medicine*, researchers in Australia and New Zealand found that sleep deprivation can have some of the same hazardous effects as being drunk. Getting less than six hours a night can affect coordination, reaction time, and judgment, they said, posing "a very serious risk."

In 1999, Eve Van Cauter, a sleep researcher at the University of Chicago, reported in *The Lancet* that lack of adequate sleep can create a pre-diabetes state in the body, which can, in turn, contribute to obesity. Van Cauter's suggestion came after a study in which six young men were allowed only four hours of sleep each night for a week. During the week the subjects were tested and found to have impaired glucose tolerance, essentially a pre-diabetes state. The sleep-obesity connection is troubling from all angles. Obesity itself impairs sleep, thus setting the stage for a scary vicious cycle.

Van Cauter also points out that two very important hormones, growth hormone and leptin, are secreted primarily during the sleep hours. Leptin is a critical hormone with respect to eating and weight management. It signals the body to stop eating carbohydrates. "With the low-leptin levels of sleep debt, your body will crave carbohydrate even though you've had enough calories," says Van Cauter.

YOUR TWO-PHASE BODY

The body's physiology basically runs on two twelve-hour phases. The time between 6 AM and 6 PM is called the *catabolic* phase. During this cycle, your body is willing to do pretty much anything to keep you up and running, meaning it is going to continually sacrifice Peter to pay Paul. Simply stated, if your left leg needs something your right leg has, your body will borrow it from the right leg and give it to the left. If your heart needs a certain raw material more urgently than your adrenal gland, the body will make sure your heart gets it, and your adrenal glands will have to make do. This process, called catabolism, permits damage to certain tissues in order to keep others with a higher priority running efficiently. But don't worry. Your body is quite smart.

Enter phase two, the *anabolic* cycle, from 6 PM to 6 AM. This is when the body repairs all the damage and borrowing that went on during the catabolic phase. The process, called anabolism, transpires primarily when we are sleeping (or should be). This is a key point. The body repairs damage through the medium of subtle energy fields that cannot be effective during the active part of the day. These fields organize the repair effort, and reach their maximum potential during sleep, particularly the deeper levels of sleep.

This is precisely why sleep is so important. *Without an adequate sleep period, people are unable to fully repair the damage they create during the day.* A chronic lack of adequate sleep results in accelerated deterioration of the body, leading to premature aging. Sleep is even more important for those who exercise and lead very active lives.

IF YOU DON'T SNOOZE, YOU LOSE

The current stress-oriented 24/7 culture isn't doing much to help people stay healthy. I love capitalism, but the daily decisions people make often reflect a greater desire to make sacrifices for money than for health, and getting enough sleep is a good example of this. In fact, for too many, the prevailing attitude has become—*if you snooze you lose.*

You will often meet people who actually brag about how little sleep they need, saying, "I can get by on only four to five hours of sleep and still exercise and have a fully productive day." While this macho attitude may be impressive, I'm sure these people have no idea how negatively it is impacting their health.

Many won't go to sleep early enough because they want to watch TV. Having been convinced by the news industry that news actually changes from day to day, they can't see going to sleep until they have been brought up to date. Nothing could be further from the truth, however. I watch the news about once every one to two months, and I can honestly tell you I miss absolutely nothing of real importance in-between viewings. Similarly, the only thing I find interesting about the late night guest shows is why anyone would prefer them over a good book.

Mr. Sandman Says . . .

※ Take your sleep time seriously.

※ Work towards getting eight hours of good, solid uninterrupted sleep in a fully darkened room, ideally before the sun comes up. If you can't do this, blacken your room or use eyeshades so it is still dark after the sun has risen.

※ Avoid food or alcohol for three hours before bedtime.

※ Lights left on in the room interfere with sleep. The production of melatonin, perhaps the single most important hormone for the immune system, occurs during sleep. It is immediately cut off by exposure to light.

Decreased melatonin production is thought to be one of the factors leading to breast cancer.

⁂ If you have to get up in the night for a trip to the bathroom, don't turn on the lights. If you need light, use a red-colored night light—red light does not seem to curtail melatonin production.

⁂ If you routinely get up to urinate, restrict your fluids before bedtime.

⁂ Chronic insomnia is a serious health problem. If you have this problem, don't think you're solving it by taking drugs. You're not. Studies show that sleeping medications interfere with the development of the deeper levels of sleep. So instead, treat the problem by following my other secrets in this book—exercise, adequate water intake, breath meditation, exposure to sunlight, and supplements, can go a long way towards relieving insomnia. Also limit or eliminate your intake of all caffeinated drinks. Certain herbs, particularly chamomile and valerian, are especially helpful to induce sleep. If you are over forty-five, try .5–3 milligrams of melatonin before bedtime.

⁂ Don't use anything electric on your bed, such as electric blankets or heating pads. These devices create an electrical field that significantly interferes with the anabolic repair process. Even when they are turned off, electric heating systems still maintain an electric field because they have transformers. That's right. Even when they're off, they're on. Just get rid of them, and get a good comforter. You'll like it better anyway.

10

Secret Three—
Sunlight

Sunlight is absolutely essential to health. Sunlight deficiency will not only seriously limit energy production, it will seriously compromise your health in other ways as well. Despite the fact that people couldn't possibly survive without it—and despite the fact that the human species evolved without the benefit of sunscreen or sunglasses—the sun has become something of a medical scapegoat. So much so, that it is almost synonymous with the deadly skin cancer called melanoma. This hysteria is unfounded.

It makes no sense at all to indict the sun for the rise in melanoma. Or, as some experts have done, blame it on the hole in the ozone layer that lets in more of the sun's ultraviolet (UV) rays. The hole is restricted to the area over Australia and thereabouts, and fails to explain the dramatic increase in melanoma *all over the world.* People have always been exposed to the sun. One hundred years ago the average exposure was much more than it is today. And yet, the incidence of melanoma has dramatically increased, even as the average exposure to the sun has decreased.

Clearly, this cannot be caused by the sun. I believe, instead, that a good deal of the increase in melanoma can be attributed to the very same factors that have brought about an increase in every other type of cancer: *Decreased energy production resulting from poor food choices, stress, and toxicity.*

In 1982, a comprehensive report by the National Research Council on *Diet, Nutrition, and Cancer* concluded that much of the rising cancer rate in the U.S. was due to the typical American diet. And, according to the National Academy of Sciences, 60 percent of all cancers in women, and 40 percent of all cancers in men may be due to diet alone. Smoking and passive exposure to cigarette smoke have also been linked to the increased incidence of all cancers, including melanoma.

It is well documented that overexposure to the sun—and the resulting sunburn—definitely increases the incidence of a type of common skin cancer called basal cell carcinoma. It is not yet known, however, whether this is any factor at all in melanoma.

What *is* known is this, and sun worshipers should pay heed: Sunburn, even a slight sunburn, does cause premature aging of the skin, including wrinkles and pigmentation. So it is advisable during the summer to limit exposure between 10 AM and 3 PM and not let yourself become burned.

Am I telling you to stay out of the sun? No, far from it. Just be cautious. There's no big secret about that. It's common sense.

My anti-aging and energy secret involves the flip side of all this, that is, the essential and positive aspects of sunlight, and just how valuable it is to your health. I am more concerned about people not getting enough sunlight, and consider this an overlooked issue.

According to the late Dr. John Ott, an expert in the biological effects of light therapy, there is no doubt that too much UV is harmful. "But the fear of ultraviolet is causing people to overprotect themselves from sunlight to the point that they are creating a deficiency of a very essential life-supporting energy."

DON'T BECOME ECLIPSED

Shut-ins, sun-shunners, and office workers run the risk of sunlight deficiency. Your doctor may not tell you this, but sunlight deficiency results in biological imbalances that will lower your energy production. It also causes a myriad of clinical problems, including anxiety, depression, hypothyroidism, insomnia, osteoporosis, and a suppression of the immune system, leading to both breast and prostate cancer.

SUNLIGHT DEFICIENCY = ENERGY DEFICIENCY

Are you getting enough sunlight? The fact that sunlight is an important factor in energy production is well established. Many studies have shown a decrease in the basal metabolism of both animals and people when they do not receive enough sunlight. The decline in metabolic rate commonly seen in everyone during the winter is a direct result of decreased exposure to sunlight. Sunlight deficiency is not usually an issue for those who live closer to the middle latitudes because sunlight is readily available all year long. But for the rest of us, it can be a big issue.

For those in colder climates, the shorter days of winter and late fall can be problematic. Bundled up from head to toe, millions leave for work and return from work in the dark. And the weather keeps them inside during the day, for weeks and even months, without exposure to sunlight. This single factor is undoubtedly what triggers flu epidemics and why they tend to occur primarily during the cold months.

Well, you may be thinking, I work in a glass-encased office building and the light comes streaming through the glass. Sorry, that's not much help. Glass interferes with the absorption of certain spectrums of UV light that are critical to the functioning of the immune system. Exposure to sunlight through windows is better than none at all, but it is of limited usefulness, and will not completely provide for your biological needs. You need the real thing—sunlight sans glass.

Sunlight exposure is also important for those who work under conventional fluorescent lights. These lights are unable to produce many of the most important spectrums that our bodies need. If possible, try to have *full-spectrum* fluorescent lighting installed. If that's not an option, be sure to get out in the sunlight.

SUN HEALING

In the late 1800s and early 1900s, a Danish medical researcher named Niels Finsen developed an ultraviolet (UV) light treatment to treat an infectious skin disease called lupus vulgaris, for which there had previously been no cure. Finsen and his successors were able to demonstrate a remarkable 98-percent success rate simply by exposing affected areas of the body to UV light. Ultraviolet refers to the radiation that comes naturally from the sun. Some man-made lamps can also produce UV, but for most people, the sun is the primary source of UV.

Finsen subsequently discovered something even more exciting. He had wondered whether the success of the treatment was due to a direct antibacterial effect of the light on the skin, or whether the results could be explained by the effect of the light on the immune system. To determine this, he treated a number of people with the disease by exposing only the unaffected parts of their skin to the light. He discovered that even when infected skin was not directly treated, the infection cleared up just as rapidly as it did for those whose infected areas he treated directly. Which is to say, the light itself was not killing the infection, but instead it was some internal physiological process that was stimulated by the light.

For his breakthrough in demonstrating the healing power of light, Finsen was awarded the Nobel Prize in physiology and medicine in 1903. The award was given "in recognition of his contribution to the treatment of diseases, especially lupus vulgaris, with concentrated light radiation, whereby he has opened a new avenue for medical science."

What Finsen did not then know was that he was stimulating Langerhans cells in the skin. These cells are vital to immune-system function. They are important antigen-presenting cells, meaning they communicate (that is, present) the infection to other immune cells. This, in turn, initiates a proper immune response.

Perhaps it is the effect of sunlight on the Langerhans cells that accounts for the most amazing of all stories regarding the use of sunlight to treat disease. Following Finsen's breakthrough research, a medical doctor named Auguste Rollier opened a sun clinic in the Swiss Alps, high above the cloud layer. Here, at Le Chalet, as he called his clinic, he developed the therapeutic use of sunlight, along with a balanced diet, exercise, fresh air, and rest, into a powerful healing-art form. This was in an era before antibiotics, and Rollier documented many impressive cures for tuberculosis and other diseases.

His patients resided in hospital rooms oriented to the sun, which had huge glass windows. In addition, each room had a balcony large enough to accommodate a bed. And, whether in beds or chairs, his patients exposed themselves to the sun for about two or three hours a day in the summer, and three or four hours a day in the winter. Rollier was convinced that sunlight combined with excessive heat had negative effects on his patients, so he did not allow them out in the middle of the day during the warm summer months. He treated his patients with this controlled exposure to sunlight during periods lasting as long as eighteen months. The results? Deformed, sick children with spinal tuberculosis were literally transformed into healthy, energetic, fully functional youngsters with straight backs, completely free of disease.

Rollier's success with tuberculosis and other infectious diseases was so significant that he established some thirty-five sun clinics from 1903 to 1940. At the height of his Alpine healing enterprise, he was able to treat more than a thousand people a day. Rollier published extensively on the curative power of the sun, reporting not only miraculous cures of tuberculosis, but also success against abscesses and bone infections. His treatments were also effective for rickets, various anemias, and a variety of non-healing wounds.

For the record, there were no cases of basal cell carcinoma or melanoma observed in any of the people he treated in these clinics. This is undoubtedly because he made sure that his patients became gradually accustomed to the sun without getting sunburned.

In recent times, the prevailing sunlight-causes-cancer bias has motivated researchers to focus on proving—in test tube experiments—that doses of UV light high enough to cause sunburn can damage the Langerhans cells. Most doctors unfamiliar with the work of Finsen and Rollier cite these test-tube studies as proof that sunlight causes cancer. In these studies, researchers exposed various human cells in a test tube to extremely high doses of an unnatural spectrum of artificial light. I have not seen one study that actually used sunlight. These experimental conditions represent exposures to light spectrums that don't exist in nature and are known to cause sunburn. It is not surprising, therefore, that the exposed cells became damaged and exhibited changes consistent with cancer and impaired immune activity. Had the researchers paid attention to the work of Finsen and Rollier, they would have learned that both doctors achieved their healing results without inducing sunburn.

Finsen and Rollier are classic examples of why you can't always translate isolated laboratory test tube findings to real life. Many times the results bear little resemblance to what happens in vivo—that is, inside the body.

To further make my point, I'll cite a study conducted by dermatologists at the University of Turku in Finland, published in the journal *Experimental Dermatology*. The researchers found that high doses of UV light could indeed damage Langerhans cells in a test tube. But when skin is exposed to UV, even high doses of it, they found that the Langerhans cells are actually up-regulated, meaning they are stimulated. This study suggests that, in reasonable doses, sunlight actually stimulates and enhances immune-system function and efficiency, and helps to explain why Finsen and Rollier were able to cure the "incurable."

I am convinced that correct sunlight exposure and a healthy diet will prevent the very same skin cancers that some say are caused by the sun.

THE SUNSHINE VITAMIN

Sunlight is the *rate-limiting* factor in the production of a very overlooked vitamin—specifically, vitamin D. The term rate-limiting means that if a necessary substance in a particular chemical reaction—in this case sunlight—is not present, then the production of the end product suffers. Your skin tissue makes vitamin D, the amount of which depends on your exposure to sunlight. Not enough sunlight results in a deficiency of D, which is why vitamin D is known as the sunshine vitamin. Some people think that the diet can supply enough vitamin D, but this is wrong. Even a diet extremely high in vitamin D cannot raise vitamin D blood levels as high as five minutes of exposure to the sun can.

The implications are immense. For one thing, as discussed in Chapter 4, vitamin D promotes the body's absorption of calcium, essential for the normal development of healthy teeth and bones. Without adequate exposure to the sun, vitamin D levels fall to a dangerously low level. A level so low that osteoporosis can result.

In 1979, the *British Journal of Medicine* published a study on the vitamin D levels of twenty-three older people followed for sixteen months. In July, they had normal vitamin D levels, but by November the levels had dropped an average of 19 percent, and, by the following February, 65 percent. At this point almost one-half of the group had levels consistent with the development of osteoporosis. This is a startling demonstration of the powerful results of sunlight deficiency.

Another common disorder associated with aging is gradual hearing loss due to otosclerosis, an abnormal growth of bone tissue in the inner ear. The growth prevents the ear from working properly. The hearing loss is sometimes accompanied by chronic ringing in the ears (tinnitus). Otosclerosis is a multifactorial disease (caused by a variety of factors), among them, a deficiency of vitamin D.

A 1985 study published in *Otolaryngology and Head and Neck Surgery* indicated for the first time that since a low level of vitamin D may contribute to demineralization of bone tissue in the ear, supplementation could help some people. Today, vitamin D is part of the medical treatment for otosclerosis. But it's my guess that if people got an adequate amount of sunlight during their lives, there would be much less otosclerosis in the first place.

SUNLIGHT AND CANCER

A commonly overlooked fact is that vitamin D is deeply involved in the way the immune system controls cancer. Although the full mechanisms of this connection are unknown, a glimpse into the possibilities is provided by a paper published in 1999 in *Cancer Research* by the Department of Medicine at Harvard Medical School. These researchers found that the vitamin D deficiency caused by an elevated calcium intake resulted in an increased incidence of advanced prostate cancer. The authors state, "Our findings support increased fruit intake and avoidance of high-calcium intake to reduce the risk of advanced prostate cancer." Other studies show the same relationship with breast cancer.

Breast and prostate cancer aren't the only cancers associated with low vitamin D production. In an amazing nineteen-year study, published in *The Lancet* in 1985, researchers found that men with the lowest levels of vitamin D (even though the levels were still within the normal range) were more than twice as likely to develop colon cancer than individuals with the highest levels.

THE PENETRATING POWER OF SUNLIGHT

Since people don't run around in loincloths, you would think clothing blocks much of the light. Most people think sunlight affects only the very outermost skin, but this is far from reality—several inches far.

To see how deeply light penetrates, William Campbell Douglas, M.D., a contemporary pioneer in the use of ultraviolet light therapy, offers a simple experiment in his fascinating book, **Into The Light.** Simply darken the room you're in and hold a flashlight under your hand. The light actually shines through the entire thickness of your hand.

How much stronger is sunlight.

Try the same experiment with some material between your hand and the light, and you will find the results are not all that different. The light still comes right through. To quote Dr. Douglas, "It doesn't take a rocket scientist to figure out that if you can see the light illuminating the top of your hand then, obviously, the light has penetrated your hand."

And that's just a flashlight—sunlight is much more powerful. It can indeed penetrate into the body, even through clothing, where it can be very beneficial, causing an increase in energy production, an increased vitamin D synthesis, and an increased functioning of the immune system.

My Recommendations to You

☀ Remember that too much of anything, including sunlight, can be harmful.

☀ The best time of day for sunbathing is during the morning hours.

☀ Start off your exposure to the sun gradually, and cover your face. Sunbathing should not include the face because it already gets plenty of exposure and excessive sun will cause wrinkles.

☀ Never expose your skin to an amount of sunlight that will create more than a barely perceptible reddening of the skin twenty-four hours later. If you are fair-skinned, this may be no more than ten minutes at first.

☀ Don't use sunscreens when you sunbathe. They interfere with the full spectrum of the light. Use them only in situations, such as in certain athletic activities, where cover protection is impractical and without sunscreen you will become burned.

☀ Wear a hat so the thin, ultra-sensitive skin of your face, head, and neck is protected. The skin in these areas receives much more exposure than other parts of the body. Protecting these areas can minimize wrinkles, age spots, and blemishes that will make you look older than you really are.

☀ If you live in the Northern or Southern lattitudes, take two or three capsules of cod liver oil per day in wintertime, just to ensure an adequate dietary intake of vitamin D. If possible, during this period of the year try to get outside in the middle of the day for at least twenty minutes.

11

Secret Four—
Supplements

For many people, one sure way to amplify energy production is to take the right supplements. And this is very individual because the need to supplement your diet is genetically controlled. Some will need much more of a given supplement than others. There are even a few who can get all they nutritionally need from a healthy diet alone. I know, I have seen them. They come into the clinic and test out beautifully on Bio-Energy Testing, despite the fact that they take no supplements at all. It can happen, but for most, this would just be a pipe dream.

It may seem like a fairy tale in this day and age, but once upon a time (not so very long ago), taking vitamin and mineral supplements was a controversial issue for doctors. The American Medical Association and many physicians emphasized that a *balanced diet* was enough to provide all the nutritional requirements for the average Joe or Jane. Many physicians even maintained that supplements could be dangerous, although there was no evidence of medical injury from their proper use.

In recent years, the tide of opinion has turned significantly. The 1990s witnessed a huge worldwide wave of scientific validation for the use of supplements, ranging from vitamins and minerals to the most esoteric rainforest herbs. Moreover, mounting consumer and patient interest has forced many doctors to rethink their attitude and modify any anti-supplement bias.

In addition, it is now widely recognized that large numbers of people don't eat a healthy balanced diet. Instead, they eat unbalanced diets heavy in processed convenience foods, thereby guaranteeing themselves nutrient deficiencies that can only lead to health problems.

Today, physicians are routinely exposed to positive articles on the beneficial aspects of proper nutritional supplementation in the *Journal of the American Medical Association* (*JAMA*) and other leading medical publications. This represents a 180-degree turnaround from the past. We now see a plethora of articles citing the many benefits of supplements, including the following.

※ How B_6, B_{12}, and folic acid help prevent heart disease

※ How chromium supplementation aids diabetes

※ How coenzyme Q_{10} rescues ailing hearts and also protects against the dangerous side effects of cholesterol-lowering medication

※ How oral magnesium tablets prevent fatal cardiac arrhythmias

※ How a simple extract of rice bran causes cancer cells to revert back into normal cells

※ How vitamins A, C, E, and the mineral selenium combat the development of cancer

Keeping up with the nutritional research is almost a fulltime job. The information is torrential. The question is no longer, "Should I be taking supplements?" The question is now, "Which are the most important supplements for me, and at what dosage?"

Proper, effective supplementation is really an individual matter, and not a matter of RDA—recommended daily allowance. The RDA represents comically minimal amounts of a nutrient and is designed only to stave off a deficiency disease, not augment health. RDA's don't take into consideration an individual's unique physiology, physical condition, size, sex, degree of exercise and activity, or environment. As such they are completely useless.

Precise nutritional needs can only be determined using some fairly sophisticated testing, along with a detailed history and physical examination. Even after all of that, it still often boils down to trial and error.

My central criteria is how well a person produces energy, since virtually any nutrient deficiency will result in a decrease in energy output. Therefore, if my patient tests out well on her/his Bio-Energy Test, I can be assured that all person's the nutritional needs are being met. Conversely, if the test results indicate poor energy production, then I know I will have to play with various supplements until the missing links are found. Having said that, there is still much that can be said in a general way about taking supplements.

PRINCIPLES OF SUPPLEMENTATION

I have been testing the biochemical and nutritional patterns of my patients for over twenty years. This experience has taught me some important general principles regarding nutritional supplementation.

First Principle

Vitamins and minerals don't work unless they supplement a good diet. *Taking supplements while on a fast-food, high-sugar, low-fiber diet is a complete waste of time and money.*

Surprised? You shouldn't be. Taking supplements and eating a poor diet is like building a house on quicksand. Even if you took a hundred supplements three times a day, it would be impossible for you to get all the nutrition you need. Every nutrient requires numerous other nutrients to be present in order for it to exert its own particular effect. Only a non-toxic, nutrient-dense, high-fiber, high-protein diet, such as I will discuss in the next chapter, can guarantee this.

Second Principle

Supplements should be taken in a balanced way. Typically, people read a magazine article extolling the virtues of a new super-nutrient, then rush out, buy the supplement, and start taking it.

Forgotten in this willy-nilly approach is that additional supplementation of other nutrients is often required to preserve the balance needed to support and bring out the effect of the super-nutrient.

Always remember that vitamins and minerals work together as a team. For example, vitamin E, the amino acid cysteine, and selenium work together to form glutathione peroxidase, a star antioxidant enzyme produced in the body. Taking one without also taking the others just doesn't make sense.

Your supplementation program should always reflect respect for balance and synergism. A broad range of nutrients, not just popping the supplement of the month, will serve you best.

Third Principle

The issue of dosage is often abused. When you increase the amount of one nutrient, you may need to increase the amounts of some or all of the others if you don't want to invite an imbalance.

The principle is this: it is best to use relatively small doses of many nutrients rather than large doses of any one nutrient. This is extremely important.

This approach is particularly valuable when it involves antioxidant nutrients, such as vitamin C. Back in the 1970s, some medical and nutritional experts declared it unproven, but today almost everybody is aware that a reduction in antioxidant defense systems leads to cancer, chronic infections, heart disease, and many other degenerative diseases.

This has led to the thinking that the more antioxidant nutrients you take, the more likely it is that the antioxidant defense systems will be enhanced. But is this true? The search to find ways to keep these systems functioning optimally continues. Is it possible to take too much of an antioxidant and minimize its effect? Greater minds than mine have advocated routine megadoses of antioxidants, especially vitamin C, as a way to improve antioxidant defense mechanisms, but are they right?

I first started to consider this question in earnest after reading an article published in the *International Journal of Biochemical Cell Biology* in 1995. The article compared megadoses, typical supplemental doses, and RDA doses of vitamin E. The researchers reached the conclusion that "Further increases in vitamin E to megadose levels did not provide additional protection from oxidative stress." This means the large doses did nothing to improve antioxidant defenses any more than the standard doses.

In another study on vitamin, C the results were the same. *The megadoses were no more effective at immune stimulation than more conservative doses.*

In these two studies, megadoses were not helpful, but neither did they produce any negative effects. However, the results of a 1983 article in *Acta Vitaminologica et Enzymologica* are a little troubling. These researchers concluded that megadoses of vitamins C and A both caused an increased destruction of red blood cells secondary to oxidative damage. Oxidative damage is precisely what increasing antioxidant defenses is supposed to stop.

In yet another study, the author asserted that "ascorbic acid (in large doses) decreases the detoxification of cyanide . . . through diminishing the availability of cysteine," and thus renders the liver more susceptible to oxidative damage. Cysteine, an amino acid, is a precursor to glutathione, a primary antioxidant and detoxifying protein in the liver. So, taking too much of one antioxidant, in this case vitamin C, ironically resulted in the depletion of cysteine, another antioxidant.

These reports prompted me to conduct a small experiment in my clinic. I divided a group of volunteer patients in half according to whether they took megadoses of vitamin C or more moderate amounts. I then infused a solution of hydrogen peroxide into their bloodstreams. I used hydrogen peroxide because it is safe, and because it is known to tax the antioxidant defenses. Blood samples were taken immediately after the infusion and analyzed for how much oxidation was present. The analysis showed that the antioxidant defenses of those on moderate doses of vitamin C was significantly greater than those taking the megadoses. I also discovered that the strongest antioxidant responses appeared to be in those who took moderate doses of vitamin C and who regularly engaged in aerobic exercise.

This study, and the others I have cited here, have convinced me that mega antioxidant supplementation is neither necessary nor desirable as a routine preventive measure. Moreover, such megadosing may, in fact, decrease the body's ability to defend against oxidative stress. The point I want to leave you with is: Avoid megadosing on your own. It is a therapeutic concept that can be useful at times, but it should only be done with the guidance of a nutritionally savvy physician.

MY SUPER IMMUNE QUICKSTART® AND SUPER FAT®

QuickStart in combination with Super Fat is the complete nutritional supplement I developed and vigorously recommend to my patients. I'll tell you why.

I have put a lot of thought and twenty-five years of experience into the formulation of this unique blend of nutrients, herbs, oils, fiber, and amino acids. While it was never meant to be a substitute for a healthy diet, I believe the spectrum and doses of QuickStart along with Super Fat reflect the current state of the art in medical and nutritional science.

I first began to make QuickStart for my own patients more than fifteen years ago, long before it was ever commercially available. The feedback I got from my patients was so gratifying that in 2000 I decided to make it available to everyone.

But here's the point. I did not write this book to sell QuickStart and Super Fat. I created QuickStart long before I wrote this book simply because there just wasn't anything comparable to it on the market. And also because I wanted to save my patients the money and time required to take all the ingredients separately.

I don't really care if you use QuickStart and Super Fat or simply take all the ingredients they contain in a separate form. In fact, in case you want to do that, I have included all the ingredients along with their doses in Appendix A. The ingredients in QuickStart and Super Fat represent my idea of a complete supplement program for everyone. Nothing has been left out, but if you decide to make your own substitute, that's fine. As long as you're happy, I'm happy.

That said, here's what it's all about. QuickStart comes in powder form. I tell my patients to use it as part of a power-breakfast smoothie that will literally give them a rocket-launch boost-off each morning.

It makes a delicious one-stop therapeutic formula that provides all the supplementary nutrition and immune enhancement most people will need. It is also designed to powerfully assist the detoxifying activity of the liver.

I haven't yet performed any double-blind clinical studies to demonstrate that QuickStart is better than any other herbal/nutrient mixtures. I just know it gets the results that my patients and I are looking for.

The reason for this gratifying effect is, the formula works on so many basic levels. It is formulated to alkalinize tissues, enhance immunity, improve brain function and circulation, increase energy production, and stabilize the appetite. *More importantly, it is specifically designed to provide all the various nutrients your liver needs to keep your body maximally detoxified.*

It is important to mention that QuickStart does not contain meaningless amounts of many nutrients just to make the label look good. Every ingredient is tried and true, and is added in its *full therapeutic dose.*

And I not only recommend QuickStart to my patients—my whole family takes it every day. It's a fabulous way to start the day.

A DOZEN REASONS TO TAKE THE QUICKSTART FORMULA*

One

It provides both preventive and therapeutic benefits.

*See page 169.

Two

It comes as a fine powder that ensures maximum absorption, even for individuals with less than perfect digestive systems.

Because of the complex nature of the digestive tract, capsules and tablets are an inferior way of delivering nutrients. Much of the vitamin content of pills is ruined in the manufacturing process. Moreover, tablets and capsules often do not adequately break down, which means that much of their content is not absorbed.

It would require over sixty large-sized capsules to pack the same amount of nutrients found in a routine dose of QuickStart. Few people will take that many pills for very long. The formula has been carefully formulated and scientifically manufactured so that each vitamin, mineral, and herb present is delivered in the most effective form. If needed for a specific therapeutic reason, other supplements, can easily be added to the mix.

Three

The formula tastes great. It mixes quickly and easily with water as a breakfast drink. Compared to pills, this is a much more natural and less complicated way to take nutrients.

Four

It's more affordable than all the bottles of pills required to get similar protection. Back in 1999, I used the catalog of a major supplement retailer to determine what the total cost of all the ingredients in a one-month supply of QuickStart would be if they were purchased separately. The results came to a tally of $163. Since QuickStart sells for $65 a container, that represents a difference of almost $100 per month. It's probably even more economical now.

Five

It satisfies the appetite and is thus beneficial as an aid for weight control. The contents are low in carbohydrates and high in energy-boosting ingredients. It is suitable for all diets.

Six

QuickStart detoxifies the liver, and restores and maintains optimal bowel function.

Seven

It contains extra chromium—a full 1200 micrograms per serving—necessary for protection against blood-sugar disorders in a society where high-carbohydrate diets are contributing to rampant diabetes.

Eight

It contains astragalus, a superb Chinese herb that enhances immune-cell effectiveness and antibody production, as well as inhibiting suppression of immune function by tumors.

Nine

It contains therapeutic doses of saw palmetto and soy isolates, shown to enhance immunity, help prevent prostate and breast disease, and regulate both male and female hormones.

Ten

A therapeutic level of ginkgo biloba helps inhibit platelet aggregation and adhesion, *and* decrease fibrinogen and plasma thickness. Translated, that means it has blood-thinning activity. Ginkgo also helps protect cell membranes, and quench free radicals. Plus, it famously improves blood circulation in the brain.

Eleven

QuickStart features a base of microfiltered, un-denatured whey protein isolate. This material is rich in antibodies, glycomacropeptide (GMP), and lactoferrin. GMP stimulates the release of cholecystokinin, a potent hormone that signals satiety to the appetite control centers in the brain, and lactoferrin binds free iron in the body, thereby reducing iron-induced free-radical production.

Twelve

The formula also benefits the heart and contains potent nutritional elements known to reduce the risk of cardiovascular disease. The unique combination of antioxidants, B_6, B_{12}, chromium, DHA, folic acid, niacin, phytosterols, and soluble fiber, improves insulin sensitivity and lowers LDL-cholesterol, triglycerides, and homocysteine levels. (*See* Appendix A for information on how to order QuickStart.)

DIRECTIONS FOR TAKING QUICKSTART

Since QuickStart is formulated to duplicate the composition of a perfect food, I recommend taking it as a breakfast replacement.

Start with a half a scoop or less. The formula is quite strong and your body may take a few days to get used to it. Add one-half teaspoon of Super Fat (discussed below) or flax oil. This is very important.

Most of my patients add extras, such as protein powder and/or fruit, but you can make it up anyway you want. Then add water or ice, according to your preference, and blend it in a blender.

When traveling, just shake it up in a container with some ice water. Don't bother with the oil on the road because it requires refrigeration. Take two fish oil capsules instead. After you've grown adjusted to a starting dose of QuickStart, gradually increase the morning dose to the recommended one scoop.

The best way to take QuickStart on work days is to take one scoop in the morning and another one in the afternoon. The afternoon dose is also very important because it will help your poor adrenal glands recover from their daily stresses.

When you first start taking the formula, you may experience a warm, prickly feeling on your neck and face. Don't be alarmed. This is just a cleansing reaction from the niacin. It will gradually disappear as you continue the program. Think of QuickStart as your breakfast, and even your lunch as well. It is an extremely good way to pave the way to high energy levels all day long.

SUPER FAT FOR SUPER HEALTH

I hope by now you are convinced that eating enough of the right fats is critically important for energy production, as well as for every single other cellular function. But from a nutritional point of view, making sure you do this can be more than a little challenging.

NINE REASONS TO TAKE SUPER FAT*

One

Super Fat is a balanced source of all the essential and non-essential poly-unsaturated fats that are so critical to health. It includes both the omega

---

*See page 169.

3 and omega 6 fats. I don't know where else you can get all these fats in one product.

Two

The essential fats in Super Fat need to be present in a particular balance for optimum results. Research has shown that the optimum ratio of the omega 6 fats to the omega 3 fats is 6:1. Super Fat maintains this ratio.

Three

Super Fat contains a supply of many of the most important, but non-essential, fats you may not get enough of from your diet. These include alpha-linolenic acid, myristic acid, octacosanol, oleic acid, palmitic acid, palmitoleic acid, squalene, and both alpha and beta tocotrienols.

Four

Super Fat is loaded with a full supply of natural antioxidants. That's very important, because polyunsaturated fats need to be taken along with the proper fat-soluble antioxidant nutrients to protect them from oxidation both in the bottle and in your body.

Five

Super Fat has the entire spectrum of vitamin-E components. These are known as alpha, beta, delta, and gamma tocopherol. This is exactly the way vitamin E is found in nature. Although most vitamins contain only alpha tocopherol, the evidence shows that the other tocopherols are equally important—research has even shown it may be unsafe to take vitamin E any other way.

Six

Super Fat contains lycopene, an important fat-soluble nutrient. Lycopene helps to prevent bladder, breast, cervical, colon, and prostate cancer. It has this effect due to its ability to interfere with the way cancers use growth factors to stimulate their proliferation.

Seven

You have already heard much about Coenzyme Q_{10}. It is critical for energy production, and is the most important intracellular antioxidant. Super Fat contains a significant dose of CoQ_{10}. It is a fat-soluble nutrient, and the fact that the CoQ_{10} in Super Fat is dissolved in other fats su[...] absorption and uptake in the intestinal tract.

Eight

Super Fat contains one of the most important of all nutrients, lipoic acid, which has the unique ability to replenish vitamin C. This is a critical reaction since humans cannot synthesize enough vitamin C for the body to be completely protected from free-radical damage. Lipoic acid is a crucial nutrient for the metabolism of fat. It also decreases insulin resistance, protects the mitochondria from damage, and is critical for optimum energy production.

Nine

Super Fat contains vitamin D_3. This is the active form of vitamin D. From Chapter 10, you know how important vitamin D is for bone health, cancer prevention, and maximum immune function.

Combining QuickStart with Super Fat and a healthy diet will provide almost everybody with all the supplementation they will ever need to produce maximum amounts of energy for all their lives. There will always be certain people, who, because of their genetics, will require higher doses, but for most this is as complete as it gets.

---

*As per federal guidelines, we need to inform you that these statements have not been evaluated by the FDA. These products are not intended to diagnose, treat, or cure any disease. If you are sick please consult a physician.

MY THREE-MONTH RULE

Every cell in your body, except the nerve and brain cells, reproduces itself within three months. This means that every three months you get to have a brand new body. If these new cells are bathed in all the nutrients found in QuickStart and Super Fat, guess what? They are much healthier cells than their parents were, and the cells produced over the next three months will be even better. This rejuvenation phenomenon will continue until you feel as good as you've ever felt. At that point continue to take one to two scoops every day for maintenance.

My Recommendations to You

☀ Supplements are there for you to improve on an already good diet. They guarantee a state of super nutrition, but they will in no way replace a healthy diet.

☀ Basically, keep it simple. Start off each day with a QuickStart and Super Fat smoothie. On work days, add another one in the afternoon.

☀ If you don't want to keep it that simple, then take a copy of all the nutrients listed in Appendix A to the health food store and get them separately. Take them in divided doses with some food.

12

Secret Five— Food

Although the right supplements can be critical for optimal energy production, a healthy and complete diet is even more so. Many times a serious decrease in energy production in one of my patients was completely turned around by simply correcting bad eating habits. This is especially true of the younger set, but it is also a big factor in all ages.

I recently read an anti-aging book that emphasized the importance of hormone replacement, supplements, and exercise. The entire discussion of food was limited to one paragraph that basically repeated the worn-out mantra of keeping fat intake below 30 percent and cholesterol intake below 200 milligrams. Giving food such short shrift does a great disservice to the reader.

Healthy eating is essential to a healthy liver, and all the hormones and exercise in the world will not make up for an unhealthy, unnatural diet. Healthy, natural foods provide essential nutrients, fats, and proteins, without which the body will be unable to efficiently produce energy.

The fact is, *today's Standard American Diet (SAD) puts the liver under siege from a barrage of antibiotics, artificial colors, drugs, food additives, pesticides, preservatives, and radiation byproducts.*

Simply limiting fat and cholesterol intake does not cut it. This information—I prefer the word *mis*information—doesn't come close to relating what eating healthily is all about.

I have great compassion for the poor consumer shopping in the supermarket. What confusion. What choices. The work of Madison Avenue reaches out with cute product names, radiant packaging, claims of fortified ingredients, and a lot of bad information to earn your purchase. In this fashion, more man-made foods have been *created* over the last fifty years than nature has produced throughout evolution. The human liver and the intestinal tract have never seen these so-called foods before. *New and improved foods* inevitably means unbalanced, man-made concoctions packed with synthetic oils and processed, fragmented nutrients—foods that are lacking in amino acids, fiber, healthy fats, nutrient balance, and trace elements. *These patented creations have absolutely nothing to do with real food.*

Whether it's a 40–30–30 energy bar or a pop tart, a much better description for these manufactured products of food technology would be industrial waste. Even real foods, milk for example, have been so industrialized they are no longer obtainable in their natural, raw state.

Unless you go out of your way to learn about real food, most of what you learn about nutrition comes from the same people who make the junk.

Confused? Sure you are.

Fortunately, I have a simple rule that can eliminate the confusion.

Shallenberger's Simple Guide to Food Selection: Don't Buy Anything With an Ingredients Label!!!

Another way of saying this is to avoid anything not made by nature. If nature made the food, it doesn't need an ingredients label. If nature didn't make it, then it isn't made for you and your liver.

Eat foods without added ingredients. That's a huge world of selection, in case you're worried. Your choices include beans, brown rice, dairy, eggs, fish, fresh vegetables, legumes, meats, nuts, oats, poultry, quinoa, seeds, unprocessed oils, whole fruit, and on and on.

A diet high in non-labeled foods will ultimately be the best one for you. Forget about simple and complex carbohydrates, fat percentage, fiber percentage, vitamin content, etc., and just choose foods based on whether there's an ingredients label or not.

O.K.—NOW READ THE LABEL

There's a slight catch in the simplicity of this concept. It's this: Not all foods have been created, or at least grown and marketed, equally. By this, I mean that many natural foods, including fruits, meats, and vegetables, are being increasingly irradiated with x-rays, and then contaminated with additives, antibiotics, dyes, and hormones. This is a big problem, especially for children. It's one thing to dose up an adult with hormones, but it's quite another to expose infants and young children to these substances.

Moreover, there is evidence to suggest that the rampant infertility among young men, and the endometriosis, menstrual disturbances, and obesity so common in young women originates largely from the estrogen contamination of beef, eggs, milk, and poultry. Fortunately non-radiated and hormone-free foods are available—look for Hormone-Free on the label.

Up to now, the FDA has not required special labeling of foods irradiated with radioactive materials. This is a travesty because irradiated foods have been shown to contain *completely unnatural molecules* that are foreign to the immune system. Since the long-term effects of irradiated foods are not yet known, I recommend they be avoided as much as possible. Unfortunately, manufacturers who are radiating foods will probably not disclose what they are doing until this is required by the FDA. Unless you grow your own food, this makes it crucial to buy your produce from sources you trust.

THE FIBER CONNECTION TO HEALTH

Humans are omnivores. That means we are designed to consume both animal and vegetable food sources. The word *vegan* is used to describe those people who, for religious or animal-cruelty reasons, among others, choose to eat only non-dairy vegetarian foods. Although practiced by a great many people who (mistakenly I believe) think it is a healthier diet, it is a highly abnormal diet. It not only doesn't make sense to be a vegan, it can be downright unhealthy. A number of studies have shown that people on vegan diets often have several deficiencies of vitamins, minerals, and amino acids. Vegans typically, though not always, test out terribly on Bio-Energy Testing. With few exceptions, they inevitably have decreased energy production.

But neither is it healthy to be a 100 percent meat eater. All life is about balance, and diet is no exception. And although animal foods contain many critical and wonderful nutrients, they do not have any fiber. You have certainly heard about fiber, and now you're about to hear more.

Dietary fiber, also known as roughage, is the portion of plant food that human digestive enzymes cannot break down. It is most readily available in beans, fruits, nuts, seeds, vegetables, and *whole* grains. Fiber absorbs moisture, acts as a natural laxative, gives the muscles in the intestinal walls something to grip on, increases in size, and makes the stool softer.

Fiber also helps to detoxify the liver. When the liver removes toxins from the blood, it excretes many of them into the intestines in the form of bile salts. Fiber, especially the soluble fiber found only in fruits and vegetables, acts like a sponge to absorb these toxic salts and escort them out of the body in your bowel movement. That's why regular bowel movements are so important to health. Without regularity, accumulated toxins build up in the intestines and the rest of the body.

But that's not all that fiber does. Much overlooked is the fact that the friendly bacteria in the intestines feed on fiber. These beneficial micro-organisms perform a wide array of services, including the elimination of harmful bacteria, and the production of vital enzymes, acids, and vitamins. Even more important, they contribute to the efficiency of the immune system. When they become depleted, your ability to fight off infections is affected.

Hundreds of studies have linked low-fiber diets to just about every condition and disease there is. These include acne, atherosclerosis, cancer, diabetes, epilepsy, gall bladder disease, heart disease, hypertension, infection, kidney stones, learning disabilities, lupus, obesity, and ulcers. There's not a lot more that can go wrong with you than that, so make sure your diet emphasizes foods that are high in fiber.

But not just any high-fiber foods. Focus primarily on the high-fiber foods that are low glycemic (see Chapter 5). This is because many of the foods that are high in fiber, such as root vegetables (tubers like potatoes and carrots) and many fruits, are also so high in sugars and other carbohydrates that they are high glycemic. And that means they create way too much insulin for most people.

The best overall high-fiber foods are those that are also low in sugars and carbohydrates. I'm talking about vegetables, specifically vegetables that grow above ground, such as broccoli, Brussels sprouts, cabbage, cauliflower, lettuce, spinach, string beans, zucchini, etc. Ideally, when you look at your plate, you should see that three quarters of it is covered with above-ground vegetables, and one quarter with animal proteins.

Although above-ground vegetables are the best source of fiber, there is no reason why most people can't also have some of the middle and high-glycemic foods, at least every now and then.

The least-desirable foods are the *refined* carbohydrate items, namely flour products and sugar. These fractured foods have very little or no fiber, and are the highest of all glycemic foods. Filling your stomach with these kinds of man-made foods is about the worst thing you can do for you health. It is an invitation to low energy and weight gain, as well as bacterial imbalance in the intestines, and increased toxicity.

One last word about flour and sweets. When you do indulge yourself, definitely avoid doing so on an empty stomach. The negative effects of these foods are maximized when eaten by themselves. Eat them only after you have already ingested some fat and protein, as with a dessert. That minimizes their insulin-stimulating effects.

FAT—MORE THAN JUST ENERGY

Whenever I start discussing diet with my patients, the first thing out of their mouths is that they are really trying to cut down on the fat.

What a great brainwashing the food industry has accomplished. Almost everybody thinks of fat as something to be avoided like the plague. The majority of the population has long been convinced, and even experts buy into it, that for the sake of health we should invest our food dollars in industrially altered food that has had the fat removed.

People are repeatedly told that fat is the enemy. And, like the cavalry, the food manufacturers are riding to the rescue and carrying low-fat and non-fat substitutes to protect everyone's health and correct the mistakes of nature.

I used to buy into this nonsense as well. Years ago, I believed that dietary fat raised blood fats and created atherosclerosis, heart disease, and hypertension. I was convinced that dietary fat was the cause of obesity. I even remember one expert who wrote that dietary fat caused diabetes.

I began putting all my patients on low-fat programs. Guess what happened? Nothing. Almost nobody lost weight. Heart disease and hypertension didn't improve, and my patients continued to complain of depressed immunity, fatigue, insomnia, and so forth.

Then I learned I was being too flexible; I was not sufficiently restricting fat. "No more than 15–20 percent of your dietary calories should be in the form of fat," came the word from the experts. So, still convinced, I clamped down and recommended that my patients eat even less fat.

Regardless of what the studies and experts say, there really is no better litmus test than patient feedback. They live in the real world, not in laboratory cages. Physicians should always keep up on the literature. But when a study leads to recommendations that just don't work with your patients, it should be ignored, and something else should be tried. That's my attitude.

Not only did my patients not improve on the low fat, but they were beginning to resent me for putting them on a diet that was extremely difficult to follow and did not taste good. The lack of results and the negative reactions caused me to do a lot of re-thinking.

I was indeed practicing medicine by placing my patients on an abnormal diet. The human body did not evolve on a low-fat diet. Anthropological studies overwhelmingly concur that the original human diet was filled with meat and fat. Studies on Eskimo Indians who actually ate nothing but meat and fat revealed a complete absence of diabetes, heart disease, or hypertension. It was only when these Indians began eating flour and sugar that they developed these diseases.

I began thinking about the diets of my patients when they first came to me, and asked myself how many obese patients ate a diet high in fat. I checked the dietary records. The answer—none.

How many of my patients with heart disease actually ate a diet high in fat. Again, none.

How many of my patients with eating disorders gorged themselves on fat? Yet again, none.

People do not develop diseases or obesity from eating too much fat. It can't be done. You can't eat too much fat even if you try. I once experimented on myself. I broiled a well-marbled steak, then covered it with butter. I quickly discovered I was stuffed before I had even finished half of it.

Compared to carbohydrates, fats and proteins sit a long time in the stomach in order to be digested. So you feel full. As I researched this further, I learned that fat induces the release of a hormone called cholecystokinin that causes the brain to rapidly register satiety. It turns out that it is literally impossible to overeat on a diet high in meat and fat. Blood sugar actually stabilizes, and many disorders of the stomach and bowels improve.

I've talked about fat as a basic energy food. But it is so much more. It is definitely something *not* to be avoided. All our cell membranes are made from fat. And over half the energy our cells produce goes into maintaining the integrity of these membranes. Research has shown that, when cells become diseased or poisoned, the very first pathological findings occur in the membranes.

Think of the cell as an exclusive club. The cell membrane is like the front door. Nothing gets in or out without going through this door. It takes proper functioning of the membrane to allow entrance into the cell of all the vitamins, minerals, fat, glucose, and proteins needed as raw materials to fuel activity. And located on the membranes are receptor sites for hormones. This is where hormones, which are messenger proteins, transfer their regulatory commands to cells. Without healthy membranes, the hormones cannot do their jobs.

Your nervous system and your brain are almost completely comprised of fats. (It is interesting to note that, although brain tissue is primarily made up of fat, the brain can only use glucose for energy because burning fat is just a little too slow for its very rapid need for energy.) Fats also serve as the building blocks for all the steroid hormones, such as cortisol, DHEA, and the sex hormones.

Fats make up prostaglandins, compounds that are intricately involved in the function of the immune system, the cardiovascular system, and the healing process after an injury.

From this, it is easy to understand why nature provided fats to eat. And why these fats should be appreciated and not avoided. Without an adequate supply of fat, people could not even begin to maintain their mental and physical health.

NOT ALL FATS ARE CREATED EQUAL

Having said this, my last statement needs to be qualified. I should say, without an adequate supply of the *right* fats. Nature has provided fats to eat, but so too has man. And once again, it is the man-made foods, this time fats, that cause enormous problems.

Take one guess as to which fats lead to decreased energy production, arthritis, diabetes, heart disease, hormonal deficiencies, immune suppression, macular degeneration, and premature aging. The answer is, the very fats the food industry has been pushing.

Decades ago, food manufacturers encountered a problem transporting and storing *processed* foods because the fats in their products quickly became rancid. In order to make their merchandise more widely available, the industry had to figure out how to get around the rancidity issue. Food scientists provided the answer in processes known as hydrogenation and partial hydrogenation. This technology altered naturally occurring fats in such a way that they did not become rancid. Moreover, these new fats were so foreign to nature that even bacteria and insects could not feed on them.

And the ideal commercial fat was created. A fat that could be stored for years without rancidity or attack from nature's predators. Food science had improved on the old-fashioned natural animal and vegetable fats, which, alas, became rancid if not refrigerated. Now there was margarine, which could sit on the countertop and thumb its nose at the oxygen in the air that causes rancidity. People could now have a cornucopia of new foods with enormous shelf life simply by using the hydrogenated and partially hydrogenated fat technology in breads, breakfast cereals, mayonnaise, and peanut butter, ad infinitum.

The only problem with the breakthrough was that these synthetic fats are alien to the body. They can't perform all the healthy functions that fats are supposed to perform. Instead, they actually interfere with the function of natural fats. They don't adequately maintain cell membranes. They adversely effect the cell-membrane receptors that are basic to hormone function. They create imbalances in the body's inflammatory response, and, in fact, increase inflammation. They block the activity of plasmin, the enzyme whose function is to dissolve platelet clots. This increases the risk of developing blood clots, which can cause life-threatening heart attacks.

Recent publications have also demonstrated that these artificial fats are contributing to cardiovascular disease by actually damaging the inner walls of the arteries. Researchers have documented that the increased consumption of margarine exactly parallels the current epidemic of heart disease. Other studies have shown that these unnatural fats change the composition of the cell membranes in the heart, and that these changes are associated with heart disease.

And worst of all, in several studies, hydrogenated and partially hydrogenated fats have been shown to damage mitochondria and dangerously decrease energy production, causing you to age faster and become much more likely to develop chronic diseases of every kind. They do this by becoming part of the mitochondrial membrane where energy production actually occurs. On the other hand, similar studies have shown that eating healthy fats actually increases mitochondrial function and energy production.

Once these destructive fats get into your mitochondrial membrane and disrupt your energy production, how long do you think it takes your body to get rid of them? On average, it takes from six to nine months of eating none of them at all to clear them all out of your membranes. These fats are poisons that take forever to get rid of, so do everything you can to make sure you don't eat them, ever.

The bottom line on fat? *Don't be concerned about how much fat you eat, just* which *fat you eat.*

HIGH FAT AND LOW FIBER

What about medical reports showing an increase in cancer among people who eat high-fat diets?

First, let me say that many of these studies are seriously flawed. Total caloric intake and the incidence of obesity are almost never taken into account. The numbers of people monitored in these studies are relatively small and the supposed increase in cancer is modest at best. Moreover, there are many contradicting studies.

For example, breast cancer is often said to be strongly associated with excessive dietary fat. In a long-term study monitoring the health and habits of 90,000 nurses, some 601 cases of breast cancer developed. However, there was no evidence of any relationship to fat intake.

In another study, published in the *Journal of the National Cancer Institute,* it was pointed out that while obesity and excess calorie intake have been implicated in cancer in both human and animal studies, fat intake per se has not. In that study, rats which had been exposed to an agent that caused breast cancer were fed either a diet high in fat but restricted in calories, or one low in fat but with a much higher level of calories in the form of carbohydrates. Only 7 percent of the rats on the high-fat diet developed breast cancer compared to 43 percent of those on the carbohydrate diet.

Unlike the supposed dietary-fat connection, when you review the medical literature, you will find many impressive studies linking deficiencies of fiber, vitamins, and other nutrients to cancer. I believe that any possible fat connection can be explained by the fact that diets high in fat often tend to be low in fiber. It is not the high fat, but rather the low fiber and deficient nutrient intake that presents a risk. Such deficiencies arise from diets lacking fresh vegetables.

PROTEIN—WHAT YOU ARE MADE OF

While fat serves the body as its primary source of energy, protein forms the structural material of most of your body. Protein is also involved in much of the biochemical business going on around the clock. Your cells need enough protein, particularly animal protein, to make muscle tissue, repair damaged organs, and produce enzymes, hormones, immunoglobulins, and brain neurotransmitters.

Unfortunately, due to the popularity of vegetarian eating, many health-conscious people have been led to believe that dairy, eggs, and meat are unhealthy for them. Additionally, since nature designed that meat and fat would travel together, the low-fat frenzy has also resulted in a decrease in protein intake.

An insufficient amount of high-quality protein in the diet has many negative consequences, including arthritis, attention deficit syndrome, chronic infections, hormonal deficiencies, immune deficiencies, low blood sugar, osteoporosis, and many other degenerative diseases associated with aging.

The preferred protein sources are dairy, eggs, fish, poultry, and meats. These can be supplemented with protein from beans and soy. For the most part, make sure you eat a significant amount of protein with every meal. And keep in mind that the more you exercise or exert yourself, the more protein you will need.

EAT LESS MORE

One of the major rules of dietary adjustment with age is to lower the percentage of calories you get from carbohydrates. The dietary carbohydrate content for most twenty- to thirty-year-olds, is often as high as 50–60 percent of the total calories. However, as you approach fifty, most will need to reduce the dietary carbohydrate content to between 30–40 percent. Additionally, since every human system is unique, some people will need to adhere more strictly to these guidelines than others. You will know how well your diet is working in several ways.

The first is how you feel. Are you as strong and energetic as always? A diet too high in carbohydrates will cause you to feel tired, especially in the afternoon. It can cause you to gain weight easily, and have a tougher time keeping the weight off. Headaches are also more common. Another manifestation of eating too many carbohydrates is in your cholesterol testing. If your cholesterol is too high, particularly if your triglycerides are greater than 110, chances are you are eating too many carbohydrates.

Of course the best way to assess your level of carbohydrate intake is through Bio-Energy Testing. If are overdoing the carbohydrates, you will test out with a low C-Factor. This indicates the degree to which your carbohydrate intake is suppressing your fat metabolism. For the same reason, you will also see a decrease in your Fat-Burning factor. And since excessive intake of carbohydrates is one of the best ways to decrease your overall energy production, you will see a decrease in your E.Q., and an increase in your Biological Age.

While you are busy getting your carbohydrate intake down, please keep in mind that, with age, fewer total calories are required. This is true even if your lifestyle and exercise level remain in a youthful fast lane. For example, a sixty-year-old man with the exact same activity level as a forty-year-old requires fewer calories to fulfill his energy needs. So, a major golden rule of eating as you age is to eat less, especially less carbohydrates, but also less fat and protein—less calories in general. Bio-Energy Testing can determine exactly what your daily calorie needs are, so you don't have to just guess about it. But in general, know that eating fewer calories is a hallmark of any program designed to keep you living longer and healthier.

THE POWER OF FASTING

As long as you are healthy, you can help keep yourself that way with regular short fasts. Animal studies have conclusively proven that fasting can significantly extend lifespan.

Basically, anytime you don't eat for two or three hours, your body begins to go into a fasting mode. Fasting, and even just skipping meals, has been shown to elevate growth-hormone levels by as much as 400 percent, a very significant result. (*See* Chapter 15, Secret Eight.)

Regular short fasting is also a superior way to detoxify the body. Many toxins, particularly heavy metals, organic acids, and substances known as advanced glycosylated end products (AGEs), become lodged in the interstitial space between cells. This is not just a domain of empty space, but is an active and systemic-wide production field where collagen is formed. Collagen is the major protein molecule that makes up the basic substance of all tissue. Collagen is what holds our blood vessels, bones, joints, and skin together. The presence of toxins in the interstitial space doesn't just interfere with the formation of collagen, it also results in a very undesirable process known as cross-linking.

Cross-linking is a general organic-chemistry term that refers to what happens when one chain of molecules is chemically linked to another one. Plastics are made through this process. And it is the effect of cross-linking that gives plastics their hard, inflexible qualities. The harder and more inflexible plastics are, the more heavily cross-linked they are. Conversly, those that are soft and pliable are minimally cross-linked. When two biological molecular chains, such as two collagen molecules, are joined through this process, they also become hard and inflexible. The result of too much collagen cross-linking is a tendency for the tissues to easily break down.

An example of collagen cross-linking can be seen in what happens to leather. Over time, even the best leather will show the classic signs of collagen cross-linking: it becomes dry and wrinkled, and ultimately cracks. A certain amount of collagen cross-linking is natural and necessary to provide structure and form to the body. It is the excess and/or unintended cross-linking that is the culprit.

Just as with the leather, when the collagen in skin and other tissues becomes cross-linked, the tissues become less flexible and less able to fulfill normal functions. The most obvious example of collagen cross-linking can be seen as people get older—wrinkles. One of the major causes of wrinkles is the collagen cross-linking that occurs as a consequence of excessive sun exposure. That's why, when you are enjoying all the health benefits of sunbathing, you should be sure to protect your face. The skin there is thin, and is very prone to collagen cross-linking.

But collagen cross-linking is more than just skin deep, its nasty effects are widely distributed. Bones will become more brittle and, as the collagen in the arteries becomes cross-linked, they will become hardened and much more likely to cause high blood pressure and strokes. The same process happens to all the organs, including the eyes, intestinal tract, kidneys, liver, muscles, tendons—everything.

Fasting helps eliminate many of the toxic molecules that contribute to cross-linking. Exercise and saunas also have the same effect, but fasting is very special in its own way. I'm not an advocate of extended fasting because there is too much protein lost from the body. Moreover, I believe the same benefits reaped from long fasts can also be achieved by a series of regular short fasts.

I personally try to get in one or two short (thirty-six-hour) fasts every month and have recommended this to my patients as well. More frequent fasting is a particularly good idea for anyone with diabetes, hypertension, or any degenerative disease process. But those with medical conditions should only fast under the guidance of an experienced health professional.

Perhaps the best way to fast is to do a daily modified fast. By modified, I mean taking in nutrients without the calories. This is an especially effective way to fast, plus it is much easier to do.

Here's what to do. Don't eat breakfast or lunch. Instead, take 1–2 scoops of my QuickStart powder along with a teaspoon of Super Fat or the equivalent (*See* Chapter 11, Secret Four). You can do this as often as you want. In addition, also drink a glass of water every hour, whether you are thirsty or not. Then, when dinner comes along, go to town. Just make sure to finish your meal three hours before you go to sleep. From a caloric perspective, this results in a twenty-three-hour fast. I do this form of modified daily fast about four days out of every week. It's easy to do, and it's a marvelous way to regularly detoxify, keep your calories down, and prevent cross-linking.

The benefits of fasting also extend to the emotional area. Even though it doesn't seem to make a lot of sense, everyone eats for many emotional reasons that have nothing to do with hunger or nutrition. People often eat simply because the regularity of timed meals confirms a sense of safety and security. As long as the meals are there, the unconscious mind can relax knowing all is well in the world. People also eat for social reasons, to squelch uncomfortable emotions, and to reward themselves for one thing or another.

For all these reasons, it is very common to confront uncomfortable feelings, such as anger, anxiety, boredom, guilt, insecurity, low self-esteem, and sadness, when going on a fast. Sometimes these emotions can be intense. They indicate the emotional connections with eating, and for many this revelation will be an eye opener. I know it was for me.

Many people either eat too much, or eat foods they know are poor choices, simply to abate current emotions. Fasting presents a wonderful opportunity to examine just how much these suppressed emotions may be running their lives without them really realizing it. And for those who like personal insights, a fast offers the impetus to deal with emotions in a healthy way, rather than continuing to suppress them under binges of chips, chocolate, crackers, or other goodies. Fasting can also instill a sense of gratitude for living in a country where hunger is rare. Gratefulness is surely one of the healthiest anti-aging emotions.

The thirty-six-hour fast I describe below represents a very manageable clean-up act. Basically, it involves not eating after 7 PM on day one, skipping food all the next day, and then breaking the fast with a piece of fruit the following morning. In addition, you'll be drinking at least a quart of water throughout the fasting day. It will be spiked with the juice of a lemon, plus honey, molasses, or maple syrup to keep your blood sugar steady. It's very simple and very effective. And it goes by very quickly. Just be sure to select fasting times that are comfortable for you, and that can fit into your schedule of activities.

MY THIRTY-SIX-HOUR FAST

First Evening

Finish dinner by 7 PM. Take 3 pancreas-enzyme capsules at bedtime, no sooner than 10 PM.

Next Day

During the day, drink at least 1 quart of pure water containing the juice of 1 lemon and a tablespoon of either honey, molasses, or maple syrup. You may drink more if you like.

Morning: Take 3 pancreas-enzyme capsules along with 1 quart of plain water immediately after you arise. A half to one hour later, take 1 scoop of QuickStart mixed in a glass of pure water, along with 1/2 teaspoon of Super Fat. Take 2 cayenne capsules and 2 acidophilus capsules with it.

Noon: Take 1 scoop of QuickStart mixed in a glass of pure water, along with 1/2 teaspoon of Super Fat. Take 2 cayenne capsules.

Afternoon (3–5 PM): Take 3 pancreas-enzyme capsules.

Dinner time: Take 1 scoop of QuickStart mixed in a glass of pure water along with 1/2 teaspoon of Super Fat. Take 2 cayenne capsules and 2 acidophilus capsules with it.

Bedtime: 3 pancreas-enzyme capsules.

Second Day

Morning: Take 3 pancreas-enzyme capsules along with 1 quart of water immediately after you arise. A half to one hour later, take 1 scoop of QuickStart mixed in a glass of pure water, along with $1/2$ teaspoon of Super Fat, 2 cayenne capsules, and 2 acidophilus capsules. During the rest of the morning eat one piece of whole fruit and drink the honey/lemon water mixture if desired.

Lunch: Break the fast with a salad.

Note: The exact doses of each of the pancreas, acidophilus, and cayenne capsules are not all that important. Your local health food store can help you.

Before or after you take the pancreas-enzyme capsules, keep a window of thirty minutes before drinking the honey/lemon water, to avoid diluting the detoxifying effect of the supplement.

You may also drink 8 ounces of coffee or 8 ounces of green tea per day if desired. You may drink as much herbal tea as you like. If you are taking hormones or medication, continue taking them as usual.

MY DIET

My patients always ask me how I eat. So, in case you are curious, too, here's the kind of diet I generally follow.

I drink a 12-ounce glass of water with a teaspoon of organic apple-cider vinegar as soon as I get out of bed.

For breakfast, I down a smoothie with QuickStart and a teaspoon of Super Fat. I shake this up with some cold water and down the hatch. On some days, I will switch up a little and make a more elaborate smoothie. To the above mixture, I'll add some protein powder and some frozen low-glycemic fruit, and blend it all in a blender. This combination is so totally balanced in nutrients, carbohydrates, protein, and fat that it is often all I have in the morning. On those mornings when I plan a long bike ride or a weightlifting workout, I will take some additional protein in the form of eggs or meat.

For lunch, I have one of several options: 1) if I'm on my daily fast, I just repeat what I had in the morning; 2) a salad with blue-cheese dressing, cheese, and meat; 3) a bowl of soup; 4) a meat sandwich; or 5) a bean, cheese, and meat burrito.

For dinner, I eat a salad, fresh vegetables, and some form of meat, poultry, or fish. I don't usually snack or eat sweets, but maybe once or twice a week I'll have a sweet or some fruit right after dinner.

My goal is to eat at least two servings of vegetables a day, and at least one fresh salad. Since every vegetable has its own unique nutrient content, I make sure to eat a variety.

I try to keep the bread, cereals, rice, and pasta to a minimum—probably no more than one to two times a week will I have anything from that list.

I am not concerned about eating too much fat or protein, and I strictly avoid non-fat or reduced-fat foods.

I eat very slowly, thoroughly chewing my food (very important for good digestion), and am usually the last one at the table to finish.

I avoid overeating.

Mornings are the most important time of the day from the angle of detoxification. That's the time to emphasize high-nutrient, fiber, and liquid intake. That's why I start my days with a lot of water and a QuickStart drink.

My Recommendations to You

❉ As much as possible, avoid man-made foods, particularly non-fat or reduced-fat foods.

❉ Avoid the regular intake of high-glycemic foods. Eat them as you would chocolate cake. I consider them strictly treat items.

❉ Limit your intake of organic coffee to 4–8 ounces a day. Too much coffee is hard on the liver, and contributes to allergies and various digestive-tract disorders. Moreover, too much java creates an acid condition in the tissues and acts as a diuretic. This combination contributes to osteoporosis because, when the level of acidity rises in the body, the system responds by pulling calcium out of bone tissue to buffer the acid. If you enjoy the stimulant effect of coffee, you might want to give green tea a try. Not only is it a strong stimulant, but it has anti-cancer properties.

❉ For these same reasons, limit alcohol to one drink a day. In small amounts, alcohol can have a beneficial stimulatory effect on the liver, as can coffee. But in excess, alcohol can cause many well-known problems.

❉ Mass-production milk has been ruined by the homogenization and pasteurization processes. Even in small amounts, it often triggers allergies in some. In larger amounts, it often causes bowel and liver problems. If you live in a state where raw milk is available, you are lucky. Raw milk has very few of the problems pasteurized milk has. (To find a state-by-state listing of raw milk suppliers, go to: www.realmilk.com/where2. html) Milk is a good source of calcium, but you can get more calcium per gram of weight from spinach and many other vegetables. *Children do not need milk at all.* Children who don't drink milk have bones just as strong as their milk-drinking friends, and they avoid the common problems associated with milk ingestion. Dr. Frank Orski, director of the Department of Pediatrics at Johns Hopkins Hospital, has pointed out that milk contributes to anemia, constipation, diarrhea, ear infections, hyperactivity, and skin rashes in children.

※ Avoid fast food, junk food, sodas, sugar, and sweets.

※ When you do eat sweets, eat them in the form of a dessert, that is, after a meal. Avoid cakes, cookies, or any sweets, on an empty stomach. By eating them after a meal, you dilute their sugar content with the other foods already in your stomach.

※ Artificial sweeteners are OK two or three times a week.

※ Use butter, lecithin, olive oil, or Pam when you cook. Avoid deep-fried foods. Learn to lightly sauté foods in a little olive oil or butter.

※ Never use margarine, shortening, hydrogenated, or partially hydrogenated oils. Never! They are poisons.

※ Forget fruit juice. It is *not* a health food. Drink juice only sparingly, as a treat. Why? It has no fiber, and is high in sugar. Did you know that a glass of most fruit juices contains as much sugar as a cola?

※ Keep your breakfasts and lunches light, and make dinner the biggest meal of the day. There may be some exceptions to this rule for those who have very physical jobs.

※ Avoid going to sleep for at least three hours after dinner. This means eating dinner early, say around 6:00 o'clock. Three hours is enough time for your body to digest the meal. If you are tired before that time, lie down and rest, but try not to fall asleep. You cannot fully digest your foods while you sleep, and this will ultimately lead to increased toxicity and weight gain.

※ Be consciously grateful for the blessing of good food you have.

※ Chew your food well. Eat slowly. And enjoy what you eat.

MY FAVORITE RECOMMENDATION

Feel free to break all the above rules periodically.

It's how you eat over the long-term that counts, not the transgressions you commit now and then. A healthy body can handle a toxic situation periodically, and besides, it gives you something different to look forward to.

13

Secret Six—
Exercise

THE MOST IMPORTANT SECRET OF ALL

First let me make this completely clear. For the over-fifty set, there is nothing you can do to increase your energy production, prolong your life, decrease your risk of disease, and slow down your rate of aging that is anywhere close to being as powerful as regular, correct exercise. Nothing. It alone sits on the throne of health.

What you eat, what supplements you take, what hormones you replace —none of these can do what exercise can do. Over the years, after doing hundreds of Bio-Energy Tests on people between the ages of fifty and ninety, this fact has become abundantly evident. Those people who improve their energy production are inevitably the exercisers. Those who don't exercise never improve. Of course the ones who do the best are those who exercise and also follow all the other secrets in this book.

But if, for some reason, you have decided to try only one of the secrets, make it exercise. It has the added advantage, by the way, of being free.

IT'S NOT FOR THE YOUNG

Few things are perhaps more misunderstood than exercise. In this country, people have the concept completely backwards. Let me explain: On the one hand, parents are almost obsessed with making sure their kids get plenty of it. They demand regular physical education classes—if you've had children in the school system, you know that getting them excused from Physical Education (P.E.) classes usually requires something akin to a letter from the Pope. Parents go to great expense to make sure that schools offer a large and diverse sports program, and they enthusiastically encourage participation.

The irony of this is, while exercise is obviously good for children and adults under thirty-five, the primary needs in these age brackets are good nutrition and adequate rest—exercise per se is not all that important. Somewhere around the age of thirty-five, however, the physiology starts to change in significant ways. And with the changes and the years, comes an increasingly greater need to exercise.

As people grow older, the metabolism levels off and begins to decline. This decrease in the metabolic rate, detectable in Bio-Energy Testing by a decreased M-Factor, is one of the most influential factors in the genesis of the diseases and infirmities associated with aging.

And it is exercise that can effectively counter this age-associated decrease. But that's not all. In the process, it also strengthens the immune system, improves cardiovascular function, increases the E.Q. (energy quotient), and significantly slows down the rate of aging.

Go into a health club, though, and who do you see? Not many seventy-year-olds. Mostly you see the younger set getting ready for their next date, while the majority of the older generation is home actively pursuing some version of couch behavior. Why? According to what I hear, most older folks have developed the idea they're too old for that stuff. Despite what they read in the popular press, which is more and more espousing regular exercise for all ages, most still don't get it. I think many people in this time of their lives just can't believe that calisthenics, jogging, and lifting weights can really do anything substantial for them. The truth is, they're not only *not* too old to do that stuff, they are too old *not* to do that stuff.

This is what I mean when I say society has it backwards when it comes to exercise. It has been accepted by most as a good way to look and feel great, but so many older people say, "I don't need to look great, and I don't feel all that bad, so why should I waste my precious time exercising?" But those who want to slow down the aging process and be fully functional as long as they live need to understand that exercise is *absolutely essential*. There is no way around it. No matter how many anti-aging hormones and supplements they take, without the correct exercise program, they are wasting their time.

EXERCISE CUTS YOUR DISEASE RATE

Aristotle said, "A man falls into ill health as a result of not caring for exer-

cise," and he was dead on. Many gerontologists (medical experts specializing in treating older people) regard exercise as perhaps the closest thing
there is to an anti-aging pill. They believe that a regular program of physical activity can go far in slowing or reversing many of the physiological
changes and illnesses associated with aging, and can thus help restore
youthful vitality.

As a longevity elixir, exercise has been the focus of an ongoing world-
famous study conducted by Stanford researcher Ralph Paffenbarger, Jr.,
M.D. With updates published over the years in leading medical journals,
the study tracks exercise habits and longevity among more than 17,000
Harvard alumni. In a 1986 report for the *New England Journal of Medicine*,
Paffenbarger said his findings show that "people who are active and fit can
expect to live a year or so longer than their sedentary counterparts. For
each hour of physical activity, you can expect to live that hour over—and
live one or two more hours to boot."

But exercise does so much more than just extend your life. It also dramatically improves the day-to-day quality of life. Here's more evidence.

※ According to Dr. Ken Cooper, M.D., of the Cooper Institute of Aerobic
Research, there are 40 percent fewer heart attacks among women who
exercise and 60 percent fewer among exercising males. In another study,
he determined that individuals in the lowest 20-percent bracket of cardiovascular fitness had a death rate three times higher than the fittest
group. The study also indicated that men who started exercising, even
after the age of sixty, increased their life expectancy.

※ Among post-menopausal women, osteoporosis can be reduced by
weight training twice a week. This increases bone density, plus improves
strength and balance, which can reduce the risk of falls in older people.
This lowers the mortality rate because fractured hips from falls are associated with a fairly high death rate.

※ A 1994 study in the *Journal of the American Medical Association* (*JAMA*)
points to a decreased incidence of gastrointestinal hemorrhage among
older people who exercise regularly.

※ An article in the *Archives of Internal Medicine* demonstrated that men
who were physically unfit were almost three times as likely to die from
all causes, including cancer, even after the researchers accounted for age,
alcohol use, and smoking.

☀ Studies have shown that exercise reduces the incidence of colon cancer by 50 percent, and of breast and ovarian cancer by a very significant margin.

☀ Impotence occurs in 25 percent of all men over the age of sixty-five. Researchers say, however, that men who regularly exercise have a much lower incidence of this problem. *If you like sex, you're going to love exercise.*

☀ Exercise is the healthiest way to treat depression. A 2000 study reported in *Psychosomatic Medicine* concluded that exercise provides as much effectiveness against depression as the latest medications—and with no side effects. Additionally, people who exercised actually had better long-term results than those on medication. After six months, those on medication had a three times greater relapse rate than those who exercised.

☀ Exercise also helps keep Alzheimer's at bay, as well as the *usual* mental decline associated with aging. It is also a very effective treatment for insomnia.

EXERCISE—IT'S ADDICTIVE

Getting sedentary people to exercise is often a challenge. Sometimes it's harder than getting them to make any other lifestyle change. But just try to get them to stop once they are into it for a few months. It is truly addicting, and improves the quality of life more than any other lifestyle habit.

ARE YOU EXERCISING TOO HARD?

Many people, especially those who find it hard to control their weight, are actually exercising too hard for their level of fitness and genetics. Often they rely on calculated heart-rate formulas that are notoriously inaccurate. If you calculate your exercise level in this manner, the odds are high that you are wasting much of your effort.

Currently, the formula that is most widely used by exercise experts to compute maximum heart rate is 208 − (.07 x age).

I'll apply that formula to forty-five-year-old Mary, one of my many overweight patients. It estimates that her maximum heart rate is 176 beats per minute. According to other standard formulas, her maximum fat burning rate (FBR) would occur at 65 percent of her estimated maximum heart rate, or 176 x .65 = 114 beats per minute, and her anaerobic-threshold rate (ATR) would be equal to .85 of the estimated maximum heart rate, or 176 x .85 = 150 beats per minute. The trainer she was going to had therefore instructed her to exercise at a heart rate between 114 and 150 beats per minute.

In fact, though, when we measured Mary's actual zones using Bio-Energy Testing, we discovered, not surprisingly, a very different picture from that predicted by the standard equations. First of all, her FBR turned out to be 95 beats per minute, not 114. And her ATR was measured at 110 beats per minute, much lower than the predicted value of 150. When she was working out in the zone given to her by her trainer, she was not only completely wasting her time, she was in fact exercising at a rate that was unhealthy and damaging for her. Let me explain.

Burning Carbohydrates Instead of Fat

Her trainer had predicted that her FBR, the rate at which she burns maximum fat, was 114 beats per minute. But Bio-Energy Testing determined that when she worked out at this predicted FBR, she was actually exercising above her ATR. This is where no fat is being burned, only carbohydrate stores. And so, for her entire exercise period Mary was not burning any fat at all. Instead of training her body to burn fat, all she was doing was depleting her carbohydrate stores.

According to the books, after exercise her carbohydrate stores should eventually be replenished by her fat stores, and in this way she should burn at least some fat. But this idea of breaking down fat stores to replenish carbohydrate stores turns out to be a bit of a myth for Mary for one simple reason. The hallmark of weight disorders is that overweight people are unable to mobilize fat stores to replenish anything. The only way an overweight person is able to replenish carbohydrate stores is by eating carbohydrates.

Since Mary's carbohydrate stores had become depleted from the way she was exercising, her blood sugar was low, and she had to immediately ingest carbohydrates in order to recover and feel well. In actuality, therefore, it's not her fat stores that are replenishing her depleted carbohydrate stores, it's her diet. All this was reflected in what she said when she first saw me, "I don't understand. No matter how hard I exercise, it does no good at all.

All I do is get sore, and I can't lose weight." I can't tell you how often I have heard this refrain.

Pain = No Gain

The reason Mary is so sore after exercise is because her trainer had also instructed her to spend half her exercise time at her supposed ATR of 150. But from her Bio-Energy-Testing results we were able to determine that her real ATR was 110, not 150. Anytime she was exercising above 110, which she had been doing for twenty-five to thirty minutes every day, she was going into lactic acidosis.

Lactic acidosis not only gives her needless pain (this kind of pain = no gain), but also causes her muscles to be sore, and increases the free-radical damage to her entire body. So, exercising above a heart rate of 110 actually prevents her from losing weight or enhancing her health. It also makes her more susceptible to disease and injury. Mary was experiencing the negative effects of overtraining. Because her trainer had been using completely inaccurate formulas to predict her exercise zone, her *entire* exercise time had been wasted.

Getting Your Zone Right

As soon as Mary completed her Bio-Energy Testing, I explained to her why she had been so unsuccessful. "You mean I have been exercising too hard for my own good?" Yes, I told her, that was the case. I then explained how research is continually showing that spending most of her exercise time at or below the ATR is the most effective way to lose weight and stay healthy—much better than the old push-it-to-the-limits approach.

Mary needed to lose fat, so I reminded her that her biggest problem was not that she had too much fat, it was that she did not have enough muscle. Whatever exercise program she went on, it would have to emphasize muscle gain. With this in mind, I started her on an aerobic program that emphasized fat-burning called interval training. I then had her alternate her interval program with circuit training (both methods are described below).

Mary only spent thirty minutes a day exercising, but this is really all anybody needs. I knew she was going to get great results because, using the other information from her Bio-Energy Testing, I had also put her on an individualized dietary and supplement program. Although the intensity of her exercise programs seemed like nothing to her after all she had been through, she did finally start to lose some weight, to the tune of one pound a week. More importantly, she was feeling more energetic, sleeping better, and losing her craving for carbohydrates.

In six months, she had lost all her excess fat, and we examined her Bio-Energy Testing results again. This time, her FBR had improved to 112 beats per minute, and her ATR had risen to 130 beats per minute. While these numbers were not yet where they needed to be for optimal anti-aging, they did demonstrate that Mary's overall program was working. Of course, her new FBR and ATR determined a different exercise zone, which she immediately began to incorporate into her exercise program.

Living in Lactic Acidosis

Many trainers accustomed to using fitness formulas instead of Bio-Energy Testing may find Mary's case hard to believe. They think it would become quickly obvious to anyone that they were in lactic acidosis, since lactic acidosis characteristically causes rapid breathing and muscle aching. But my research has shown me that a large percentage of people, particularly those with weight-control issues, have trained their bodies to be so used to lactic acidosis that they don't usually develop these symptoms.

Because their E.Q. is so low, they may spend a considerable part of their day in lactic acidosis simply from everyday exertions, such as walking. Some of my patients go into lactic acidosis simply from getting out of a chair. The livers in these people have often developed an extraordinary ability to convert lactic acid back to blood sugar with incredible efficiency, allowing them to be in lactic acidosis without having the characteristically severe symptoms.

Mary was one of these people. Under the advice of a trainer who used the standard formulas, she had regularly been exercising in lactic acidosis for more than two years. Exercise was not fun for her, and she had to force herself to do it. She was chronically tired and achy, but because her doctors could find no reason for these symptoms, she had just learned to live with them. Eventually, she had even stopped complaining about them.

Being in the Zone Is Fun

Not long after Mary's Bio-Energy Testing discovered her correct zones, she called me up complaining about her new exercise program. "This is much too easy," she said. "It can't possibly work. I'm sure I'm wasting my time." I assured her this was because for the past two years she had been overdoing it, and naturally it felt too easy. I told her to enjoy the fact that she would no longer have to dread her exercise periods, and she would actually begin to look forward to them. Exercising in the correct zone is fun and enjoyable. When she came to the clinic two months later, she was smiling and finally seeing the light. This was the first non-dieting weight loss she had ever seen.

Mary's case exemplifies the importance of exercising in your real zone, not an imaginary one deduced from one-size-fits-all formulas. I have seen so many cases like Mary's over the years that I often wonder if these formulas actually work for anyone at all. Knowing your *real* FBR and ATR are invaluable keys to getting the most from your workouts.

In twelve months time, Mary's numbers became optimal, and she settled into an easy maintenance program consisting of exercise for twenty to twenty-five minutes three to four times a week. She will be doing this the rest of her life, and at the rate she is going, that should be a really long time.

YOUR OPTIMUM EXERCISE ZONE

One of the beauties of Bio-Energy Testing is that instead of having to rely on an erroneous calculated formula, it is able to determine your real exercise zone. This is important, so let me just repeat myself. When you are exercising above your ATR for longer than a few minutes, your body will increase its level of free-radical damage, and it will actually age faster. When you are exercising at a level of exercise that is below your FBR, your exercise will be inefficient, and you will be wasting your exercise time. *So, whenever you exercise, be sure to wear your heart-rate monitor, and keep within your ZONE.*

There are two basic ways to exercise that really work. One is called *interval training,* and the other is *circuit training*. Interval training emphasizes increasing both your ability to burn fat and your total aerobic energy-producing capability. Circuit training accomplishes both of these goals as well, but also adds the element of resistance training to increase muscle gain. Both are valuable, and I generally recommend that each be done on alternating days. I'll talk about interval training first.

Interval Training

Interval training involves alternating longer intervals of time at your FBR with shorter times at your ATR and very brief spurts above your ATR. The time spent at your FBR is called your recovery time. It is where your mitochondria can recover from the more intense exercise you are doing the rest of the time. It is also where you will train your body to burn fat more efficiently.

A typical interval-training session begins by exercising hard enough to raise your heart rate up to your FBR. This is a warm-up period. After a few minutes warming up, start exercising hard enough to bring your heart rate up to your ATR, and leave it there for one to two minutes. How long depends on what you feel like doing. If you are having a peppy day, go for the longer time. If not, take it easier.

Next, go all out for twenty to forty seconds. This is called an *anaerobic burst* because during it your heart rate will climb way above your ATR, and you will be producing energy anaerobically—without oxygen. Although I have told you that exercising above your ATR is bad, I am now going to fine-tune that statement.

It's true. Extended time spent exercising above your ATR is harmful. Athletes need to do it to win races, but nevertheless it is not good for their health. However, brief spurts of exercise in this zone—no more than twenty to forty seconds—is actually quite stimulating for the mitochondria.

After this short anaerobic burst, your heart should be pounding, you should be breathing very hard, and you should be really happy that you don't have to do it any longer. At this point, decrease the pace to almost nothing until your heart rate comes down to your FBR.

Once you reach your FBR, adjust the pace so you stay there until you feel recovered. By this, I mean that you feel your body has recovered from that anaerobic burst, and you are ready to do it all over again. Just to give you an idea, most people need at least three to five minutes to recover. After a few intervals, towards the end of your exercise time, you may very well find that it takes longer to recover. However long it takes, just remember this: Your recovery period is *every bit as important* as is the ATR interval and the anaerobic bursts. It may feel easy, and you may think it's a waste of time, but it isn't.

As soon as you feel recovered, then repeat another interval of one to two minutes at your ATR followed by an anaerobic burst. Continue repeating the cycle of three to four minutes of FBR followed by one to two minutes of ATR, and twenty to forty seconds of an anaerobic burst. I guarantee that you will love this form of exercise. It changes enough that it's not boring, and it is so much easier than continually overtaxing your body's reserves.

Many people erroneously think the only good form of exercise is hard and fast. That may be a great way to win a race, but it is not the best way to stay healthy. It is very important to always exercise in intervals, spending time at both your FBR and your ATR. Although it is easier than spending your entire exercise time at your ATR, interval training is much more effective than any other form of exercise. It is also healthier, not to mention more fun.

Circuit Training

Circuit training involves the use of multi-set, high-repetition, non-stop weight-resistance training. It's easy to do once you learn, and it has the advantage of strengthening and building all the muscles in the body, while at the same time offering an aerobic workout.

The first thing to do is get a personal trainer to instruct and follow you for the first few months. Have the trainer set up a circuit of resistance exercises for you that work all the major muscle groups in your body. Make sure to show your trainer the instructions below. The weight-lifting movement should be slow, to avoid injury. In circuit training, the weight resistance is set so you can just barely lift the weight fifteen times.

The procedure goes like this. After you put on your heart-rate monitor, perform the first fifteen repetitions. Check your heart rate. If it is below your ATR, immediately go on to the next set, and check your heart rate again. Keep on doing this until your heart rate is above your ATR. Once this happens, sit down and rest. You can read a magazine while you are waiting. I like to answer my e-mail then.

As soon as your heart rate has come down to your FBR, start the next set of exercises. Keep on exercising in this pattern—going on to the next set when your heart rate has not exceeded your ATR, and resting when it has. Do this for thirty minutes, and your exercise is over.

MY 5–10 RULE

How many times have you arrived at your regularly scheduled exercise program only to find you just don't feel up to it? I don't know about you, but this happens to me almost all the time. My inner voice is rebelling: "I'm too tired," or, "I just don't feel like it right now."

A long time ago, I decided I had to develop a way of dealing with this in order to pursue any semblance of a regular exercise schedule. So I came up with what I call my 5–10 rule. It works for me. See if it works as well for you.

☀ No matter how you feel, start your exercise—no excuses allowed—just do it.

☀ If, after five minutes, you actually feel worse than you did when you started, you get to call it quits for the day.

☀ If, after ten minutes, you don't feel better than you did before you started, you can also stop.

I can honestly tell you that when you use this yardstick you'll rarely end up quitting. It just reaffirms in my mind the incredible value of exercise on both the physical and mental levels.

My Recommendations to You

☀ Ideally, obtain Bio-Energy Testing through your physician or at a health spa. (*See* Resources in back for a Bio-Energy-Testing expert in your area.) Determine your FBR and your ATR. Your optimal exercise zone is between these values. Unless you plan on serious competition, there is no benefit in exercising harder than described above, and there may be several disadvantages. Similarly, exercising below your FBR will yield relatively little benefit.

☀ Purchase a heart-rate monitor from a sporting goods store. You can buy a good device for about $50. Use it every time you exercise.

☀ Find a personal trainer to work with for the first six months. This is very important for your success. Go on and spend the money. It's not that much, and you are definitely worth it.

☀ If you don't have Bio-Energy Testing available, a good estimate of your ATR is that it is the heart rate at which you start becoming breathless. If you are on the treadmill, for example, start gradually increasing your speed. After a while you will start breathing more rapidly—enough so that you can't talk on the phone without the listener noticing. At this point, look at your heart-rate monitor. The reading is close to your ATR. Multiply this estimated ATR by .80 to guestimate your FBR.

☀ If you need to lose weight, exercise for at least thirty minutes every day. Alternate between interval training and circuit training, and follow the instructions in the book. If you don't need to lose weight, exercise for thirty minutes four or five times a week at your ATR, using either interval or circuit training.

☀ Also be sure to check your Bio-Energy-Testing values at least once a year. The chances are, as you get in better shape, both your FBR and your ATR are going to change.

14

Secret Seven—
Breathing Right

Breathing is elemental—like eating. You do it or else. Obviously, since breathing is how we get oxygen, poor or incomplete breathing will dramatically affect energy production in a way that nothing else can.

Contemporary science has provided the details of the gas exchange that occurs in the breathing process, but ancient thinkers put attention on this issue long before anyone had such detailed understanding. The ancients quite naturally reasoned that since *not* breathing was synonymous with death, breathing itself must be pretty important. They furthermore concluded there must be both proper and improper ways to breathe.

It turns out this is very true. There is a right way and a wrong way to breathe. And all too frequently it is done the *wrong* way. After years of seeing people diagnosed with problems, such as chronic anxiety and panic disorder, I am firmly convinced that many of them result from improper breathing. It is, in fact, a major—and widely ignored—cause of anxiety, low energy, panic attacks, premature aging, and overall stress.

MANNY'S PROBLEM AND THE SOLUTION

Shortly after I began routinely using Bio-Energy Testing in my clinic to examine the energy status of my patients, it became very clear that many of them were shortchanging themselves, from an energy standpoint, because of the way they breathed.

A primary example was Manny, a forty-three-year-old man who made his living installing dry wall. In order to be successful in a very competitive field, he worked hard for long hours. He first consulted me about low energy and

201

episodes of panic attacks. His previous doctor had told him that his tests were normal, and that the drop in his energy level was caused by his anxiety.

When the panic attacks occurred, Manny felt as though he could not catch a complete breath. His heart would beat rapidly, and he would become fearful of passing out. These episodes occurred suddenly and without warning. Although he had stopped drinking his daily pot of coffee, the problem persisted.

He was soon prescribed an anti-depressant medication. When that didn't work, he was told to work at a less stressful occupation. Since this wasn't going to fly, he came to our clinic looking for another answer.

His Bio-Energy Testing revealed a fairly significant decrease in his M-Factor (his resting energy production). The test also showed that an insufficient delivery of oxygen at the capillary level was causing this. During testing, we noticed that his respiration rate at rest was between fifteen and eighteen breaths per minute. That is way too high. A normal resting breathing rate is less than ten.

Most importantly, Manny breathed by expanding his chest, even when lying down. This is fairly unusual because most people automatically breathe with the abdomen while they are lying down. Breathing with the abdomen is known as **diaphragmatic** or **abdominal breathing** (I'll stick with the latter term). When we asked him about it, Manny said he didn't feel short of breath. He said his breathing seemed normal to him.

Immediately following the test, my technician spent a half-hour with Manny teaching him some proper breathing techniques. When his Bio-Energy Testing was re-examined afterwards, his respiration rate had come down to under twelve breaths per minute. Along with this, his energy production had increased 20 percent, to an almost optimum level.

This turnaround had occurred in less than an hour, simply because Manny had started breathing properly. The most significant development, however, came later in the form of decreased feelings of anxiety. After three weeks of continuing his breathing exercises for fifteen minutes twice a day, Manny's anxiety symptoms completely disappeared, and he had his energy back. It's amazing what can happen when causes are treated instead of just symptoms.

Such dramatic results, and in such a short period of time, show just how powerful an influence breathing habits can be. Manny's problem was not all that unusual either. Like a great many people, especially those with chronic anxiety, he was a chronic chest-wall breather, and this method of breathing aggravates, and most times causes, chronic anxiety.

THE RIGHT AND THE WRONG WAY TO BREATHE

There are basically two different ways to breathe.

Chest-Wall Breathing

Chest-wall breathing uses the chest, neck, and shoulder muscles to lift up the chest in order to inflate the lungs. As you inhale, the chest expands. The abdomen is sucked in.

This is the classic *chest out, abdomen in* form of breathing taught in the military and reinforced all throughout youth. To determine if you are a chest breather, just sit and rest quietly in a chair, breathing easily, and observe how your chest and abdomen move when you inhale. If your abdomen does not go out every time you inhale, and/or if your chest expands, you are chest breathing. This is not the preferred style.

Abdominal Breathing

If your abdomen goes out when you inhale and your chest remains still, this is abdominal breathing. Instead of raising your chest up to draw in air, military style, you are pulling out the diaphragm muscles in your abdomen to draw in air. This is the preferred style.

THE SHORTCOMINGS OF CHEST-WALL BREATHING

Chest-wall breathing fails to draw in as much oxygen to the lung's air sacks as abdominal breathing. Here's why: The lungs have what is known in pulmonary physiology as dead space. This refers to the space taken up by the tubes (airways) through which the air passes en route to the lung's air sacks, where oxygen is delivered to the bloodstream. These airways leading to the tubes are called dead space because they don't participate in the actual exchange of oxygen.

Dead space is more prevalent in the upper part of the lungs than the lower, and chest-wall breathing selectively fills the upper part of the lungs. This means that when you chest breathe a greater proportion of your breath is being wasted in the dead space. Abdominal breathing, on the other hand, selectively fills the lower part where there is less dead space, and thus greater oxygen acquisition.

In order to make up for the decreased amount of oxygen acquired per breath, chest-wall breathers automatically compensate by increasing their respiratory rate. Before Manny's breathing was reorganized, his rate at rest was typical of this—fifteen to eighteen breaths per minute. By comparison, an abdominal breather usually needs only six to eight breaths per minute to acquire the same volume of oxygen.

Chest-wall breathers are obviously working harder to acquire the same amount of oxygen as abdominal breathers. But that's only part of the downside. The other part stems from the fact that every time you breathe, you exhale carbon dioxide. Thus, if you're breathing fifteen times a minute, you are exhaling two times more carbon dioxide than when you breathe seven times a minute. This condition can be easily detected by Bio-Energy Testing because it results in an excessive excretion of carbon dioxide.

The excessive loss of carbon dioxide shifts the pH (acid balance) of the blood into a state called *alkalosis*. This has immediate and dramatic effects on the brain, often leading to an edgy, anxious sensation. Try it yourself. Take just three or four rapid deep breaths, and you will feel the difference. When people do this all the time, the condition is known as *chronic subacute hyperventilation*. This condition often leads to panic attacks and chronic low-level anxiety. Because of its effects on the blood pH, it also results in a decreased oxygen delivery to every cell in your body. Let me explain how.

When you breathe in oxygen, it gets taken up by the hemoglobin molecule contained in your red blood cells. Hemoglobin has an incredibly strong attraction for oxygen. It holds tightly to the oxygen as it passes though the arterial network and down to the level of the cells, where the oxygen is finally delivered to the cells. The hemoglobin molecule is triggered to release its oxygen cargo in response to the acid pH it encounters at the cellular level. However, when the normal acid pH becomes disrupted due to the alkalosis caused by chest-wall breathing, the hemoglobin molecule is effectively prevented from releasing its oxygen payload. The result is a decrease in available oxygen to the cells, and a decrease in energy production.

If you have ever gone through a very stressful period (and who hasn't), you may have noticed that afterwards you feel drained and fatigued. One reason for this is that stress almost always puts people into a chest-wall breathing mode, which, as noted, contributes to low energy through the alkalosis effect.

Since your body is designed to operate more efficiently through abdominal breathing, you might wonder why chest breathing evolved at all. The answer lies in the unconscious, primitive part of the brain that regulates breathing. Under emergency situations, in times of danger, the body requires additional oxygen. In the distant past, you would have needed a major injection of oxygen to flee from a lion that had you in mind as its next meal. To meet such threatening challenges, the body kicks into a double-breathing mode—chest wall combined with abdominal breathing. This sucks in a quick oxygen increase. In intense situations like these, where exertion is at an ultra-peak level, alkalosis does not occur, and oxygen uptake and delivery are maximized. The body evolved the capability of chest breathing as a survival mechanism.

Although survival and escape from life-threatening predicaments may not be part of daily existence for most, the everyday variety of mental stress so common to life today is often enough to switch on the chest-breathing response. The unconscious part of the brain reads the stress reaction as a sign of an impending emergency and triggers a subtle but slightly increased breathing rate. You may just be sitting in your car knowing you are running late for an appointment when, whamo, quite suddenly your body goes into that emergency mode. You may then experience a panicky feeling, which is all the more stressful because there is no apparent reason why you should have such a reaction. At times such as these, it becomes that much more important to make sure you are breathing from your abdomen.

THE NITTY-GRITTY ON SIGHING

Before closing the case on chest-wall breathing, I'd like to make a few comments about sighing. Although you may associate sighing with the sight of a heart throb, or another romantic imagery, the body has other primary reasons in mind.

A sigh is a distinct physiological event characterized by a deep full breath, using both abdominal and chest-wall breathing. Sighs occur naturally about every ten to fifteen minutes, allowing the lungs to completely fill up. When you are *not* exerting yourself, you use very little of your lung capacity. At these times, the body creates the sigh response—a quick, deep breath—to help expand and engage areas of the lungs not being used.

You've probably had many occasions to notice the wonderfully relaxing effect of a sigh. It often seems to automatically occur when you are stressed. The problem with chronic chest-wall breathing is that, due to its associated hyperventilation and alkalosis, the body is often unable to sigh. When this happens, it can be very disturbing.

Sometimes, a person who desires the calming benefit of a sigh, but can't do it secondary to chronic chest-wall breathing, will call me quite concerned and say, "I can't get a deep enough breath, and I think something must be wrong with my lungs." Of course, the mere thought that something is wrong with their lungs is enough to agitate most people and perhaps trigger an anxiety attack. At times like these, I just tell them to relax, and explain some basic facts on sighing to reassure them their lungs are really OK.

The first fact is, you can only sigh a maximum of once every ten minutes. Second, you can't force a sigh. You just have to be patient and wait for it to happen. Third, not being able to initiate a sigh at will does not indicate there is any problem with your lungs.

Don't be nervous if you can't sigh on demand. Just be patient and wait. It will come soon enough, but only to the degree you are breathing with your abdomen.

BREAKING THE VICIOUS CYCLE

By now, it's obvious that chronic chest-wall breathing generates a vicious cycle with a number of negative results.

* Decreased oxygen uptake in the lungs, leading to

* Decreased oxygen release to the cells, leading to

* Decreased energy production, leading to

* An emergency mode in the body, leading to

* Feelings of tension, leading to

* Increased respiration, leading to

* Interference with the sighing mechanism, leading to

* Decreased oxygen uptake in the lungs

All these promote even more chest breathing. And, as this progresses, you can readily see how an anxiety attack can develop.

When anxiety becomes chronic, most people will run to the doctor and get a prescription for a sedative. The medication slows down the respiratory rate and seems to correct the problem. However, the sedative only takes care of the symptoms, and does not correct the root problem. Even more damaging, it often creates new problems in terms of side effects.

A healthier way is to teach yourself to breathe with your diaphragm. The information below tells you how to do this. The alternative is to continue the habit of chest-wall breathing, which is just going to deprive you of optimal energy and age you faster.

HOW TO BREATHE THE RIGHT WAY

Diaphragmatic breathing is one of the very first techniques that singers and musicians are taught in order to provide them with ample oxygen for those long notes. I learned the method years ago in a yoga class and it gave me a significant advantage later when I was actively involved in competitive cycling.

The technique is quite simple, but you may need guidance because it is somewhat subtle. Once you've got the idea, it just takes a little practice over a few months to fully perfect it and make it automatic.

When I started learning the technique, I made up little signs saying "Breathe!" I put them everywhere—on my bike, my dashboard, my mirror, my watch. The signs were reminders to check how I was breathing. And when I checked, I was usually breathing with my chest. I would just take a few good abdominal breaths and try to concentrate on breathing this new way as much as possible. The other thing I did, which helped enormously, was to spend a few minutes every morning and evening performing breath meditation.

Here are a few simple points to learn the diaphragmatic technique. Many people can grasp the basic movement within a few minutes.

※ Lay down on your back. It's hard to chest-wall breathe while lying down. Even the most die-hard chest breathers tend to breathe with the diaphragm in this position.

※ Now place your hand on your abdomen. Notice how it rises slightly when you inhale, and goes down when you exhale. This movement is the hallmark of breathing with your diaphragm. If you breathe with your chest, your hand will not elevate during the inhale, it will drop down instead. If you are naturally breathing with your diaphragm while lying down, you are well on your way. If it isn't coming naturally, don't worry. Just give it a bit more time. You'll get it soon enough.

※ After a few moments of doing the diaphragmatic breathing, you become familiar with it. At that point, while you are still lying down, I would like you to exaggerate the breathing pattern by contracting your abdominal muscles inward (sucking in your gut) as you exhale the air from your lungs.

※ Then expand the same muscles outward to inhale.

※ Keep practicing this technique until you can breathe fully without moving your chest.

※ If the movement doesn't come easily, ask your spouse, or a friend, or yoga instructor to help you.

※ Once you have learned to do this lying down, try the same thing while sitting in a chair, and then while standing. Finally, to perfect your newly discovered talent, try doing it while you are singing in the shower or lightly exercising. You can then proudly announce to friends and family that you have finally learned to breathe correctly.

There are additional benefits to abdominal breathing that should inspire you. One is that it often helps the neck pain and tension commonly caused by chronically raising up the chest during chest-wall breathing. Abdominal breathing does not create any neck and shoulder strain since it moves with gravity instead of against it. It also strengthens and tightens the abdominal muscles. And finally, it often benefits those with asthma or other lung conditions.

BREATH MEDITATION

Perhaps nothing is as powerful as the mind to either make you sick or keep you healthy. But how do you learn to harness and direct that power? One tried-and-true method is breath meditation.

This meditative exercise is particularly effective for hypertension, insomnia, and other stress-related disorders. It will also generate more energy and stamina. In addition, it's a very effective way to train your mind to work better for you. That means increased clarity, memory, and speed. Another bonus is that breath meditation is completely devoid of side effects. And, there are no gyms to join or pills to take. The little time it takes to do it can lead to many wonderful rewards.

First, it's a good idea to get the concept straight. Meditation, at least the way I'm using the word, refers to mental exercise. Meditation and prayer are not the same thing. Praying is a different concept. It has its own powers, but does not substitute for meditation. So even if you regularly pray, please be sure to practice some form of meditation as well.

Breath meditation trains the conscious mind to focus better and the unconscious mind to relax better. It works the same way that training your muscles makes them function better.

Most of the time, your meditation session will be relaxing. But there can also be days in which emotions or stresses may preoccupy your mind, and you may find yourself expending more effort to meditate. You don't need to worry about that. It's normal. Just take it as it comes and apply the simple guidelines I'll be giving you. What's important to understand here is that no matter how relaxing a meditation session may or may not be, it will still serve to improve your overall relaxation potential and strengthen your powers of concentration.

Your mind is like a puppy. It wants to wander around and experience everything it can. This is a wonderful thing, but it can also limit the mind's ability to focus. And mental power is directly related to focus. Breath meditation trains your mind to focus better, and in so doing, it strengthens your mental power. This, in turn, increases the ease with which you do everything.

The process takes fifteen to twenty minutes, and if you can do it regularly, once or twice a day, it may be the most productive fifteen or twenty minutes of doing nothing you can possibly imagine. Just follow these easy steps and you'll be on your way.

Step 1—The Setting

You ideally need some quiet space, a room where you can meditate without interruptions. If there's a phone in the room, pull out the plug.

※ You need a comfortable chair, one with arm rests if possible.

※ Sit comfortably in it. Don't cross your legs.

※ Take three deep relaxing breaths, and when you exhale the third time, let your eyes close.

Step 2—Breathing in Squares

⁂ Use the abdominal breathing technique you just learned. I want you to breathe in squares. By that I mean pausing to hold your breath at the end of both your inhale and your exhale. The pauses should be the same length of time you use to breathe. For example, if you inhale (expanding your abdomen in the process) over a two-second period, hold your breath for a two-second pause before your begin to exhale. Then exhale (sucking in your abdomen) over a two-second interval. At the end of your exhale, pause for two seconds before you begin your next breath. If you inhale over a three-second count, then just make sure the other intervals are three seconds long.

⁂ Keep repeating this process for each and every breath. It's as simple as that.

You can count the seconds to yourself as go along, but after a while you will probably find you are able to naturally keep the intervals the same without counting. Just remember to breathe only with your abdomen. Keep your chest free of movement. While you go through this routine there are several things you should be aware of.

Sighs and yawns

As mentioned above, most people experience the need to sigh about every ten minutes. During meditation, when you feel the urge to sigh, just go with it. Remember that sighing invokes both chest wall and diaphragmatic breathing. After the sigh, simply return to the abdominal breathing in squares. Sometimes you may feel the urge to sigh, but it just doesn't develop. This just means your body doesn't need one yet. Sighs are relaxing, but don't force them. Be patient. One will come along soon enough.

Don't be bothered by yawning. I can remember many times when I have yawned more than twenty times in a meditation session. Just go with it, and as soon as the yawn passes, simply return to abdominal breathing in squares.

Altering your breathing rate

One thing sure to happen during breath meditation is that you will need to alter your breathing rate to accommodate how your feel. If you feel breathless while you are pausing at the end of exhalation, you will need to increase the rate. When you notice this, simply up your breathing rate by decreasing the pause length until you are comfortable and no longer feel in need of air.

As the session progresses and your body becomes more relaxed, you will usually need to decrease your breathing rate. If you start to feel a little dizzy, like you are hyperventilating or breathing too fast, just decrease your breathing rate by increasing the pause length. You may have to adjust your breathing rate a few times during a session in order to keep feeling comfortable.

Step 3—Training the Puppy

A crucial part of breath meditation is your mental focus. While you are just sitting there comfortably using your abdominal muscles to breathe in squares, it is important to keep your mind entirely focused on your breathing. You can focus on your breathing rate, how the air feels in your lungs, or how your abdomen feels as it moves in and out. It doesn't make any difference exactly what you focus on, as long as it has something to do with your breathing.

But the mind is like a very inquisitive and active puppy. It may not always reconcile itself with the drill called meditation. Imagine having a puppy on a leash and training it to sit comfortably by your side. As soon as you place the puppy on the floor next to you, it will immediately begin to wander in one direction or another. Without becoming upset—after all, you are only training it—just gently retrieve the puppy and put it next to you again.

Your mind is going to stray the same way. No matter how hard you try to keep your attention on your breathing, your mind will wander off into this or that thought. And, as with the puppy, the minute you become aware that your mind is wandering, gently retrieve it and refocus on your breathing.

This repetitive cycle of concentrating, straying, and refocusing again is the nature of breath meditation. The more you practice this retrieving and refocusing, the stronger your power of concentration will become. After several months of regular practice, you will begin to notice that your mind is wandering less, and you are retrieving your awareness more easily. Although your mind can be an extremely stubborn puppy, it will eventually learn.

Breath meditation contributes to a longer, healthier, more enjoyable, and more productive life. People who continue meditating in this fashion see an improvement in almost every health function measured. Don't underestimate the power of this simple way to enhance your mental speed and concentration, improve your mood, sleep, and emotional state, and increase your energy levels.

My Recommendations to You

☀ During the day, and especially when you exercise, check your breathing regularly to see if you are breathing correctly. Be patient, and keep working at it. It took me about two years before I was consistently breathing correctly without thinking about it.

☀ Make it part of your daily routine to practice breath meditation fifteen minutes once or twice a day as your schedule allows. The best time for most people is before and after work. At first, it may seem a little intimidating, but after a few months you will actually prefer it over any previous thing you might have done to unwind and relax.

15

Secret Eight—Bio-Identical Hormonal Replacement

I t would be impossible to discuss the topic of optimal energy production without discussing bio-identical hormonal replacement. This is because mitochondrial function is intimately tied to hormonal stimulation. In the absence of adequate hormonal encouragement, the mitochondria will just sit around and do the minimum.

Normally, when people think of hormones, they think of the sex hormones. They tend to think of hormonal replacement as something the older crew needs. And this is generally true. But many young people, as well as their older colleagues, have undiagnosed deficiencies of thyroid hormones. As you will soon see, there are no hormones more critical to energy production than the thyroid hormones. For this reason, when we doctors think of optimal energy production, we immediately think of hormones.

Undoubtedly the single most important contribution to the new explosion of anti-aging medicine has been the availability of natural *bio-identical* hormones, and the growing research regarding their effects. *The efficacy of all of the secrets I discuss in this book is greatly limited in the absence of proper hormonal replacement.*

Ever wonder how it is that young people can get away with everything? They can eat terrible diets, experience huge amounts of stress, fail to get enough rest, smoke, and otherwise carry on, and still do better than older folks on a health program. Well, wonder no more—it's all about hormones. Youth is a time of boundless levels of hormones. And as people navigate through the years, their hormone tanks become drained.

Refilling the tank has become an exciting new frontier in medicine which I am thrilled to be part of. And refilling the tank—replacing drained hormones—often produces such startling reversals in energy production and overall health that people can't believe all the good things that are happening to them. This conversation is not just limited to the significant benefits gained by restoring deficient levels of estrogen or progesterone for menopausal women. I am talking about the replacement of many different hormones in both women and men as they get older.

Here are some of the improvements experienced as a result of this approach.

※ Better mood and sleep

※ Built-in resistance to illness and infections

※ Enhanced healing

※ Enhanced sexual performance

※ Fat loss *without dieting*

※ Fortified brain, heart, kidneys, liver, spleen, and other organs that atrophy with aging

※ Improved cardiac function

※ Increased exercise capacity

※ Increased mental function

※ Increased muscle mass *without exercising*

※ Lower blood pressure

※ Lower LDL cholesterol, the bad cholesterol that contributes to harmful plaque when it becomes oxidized

※ Reduced wrinkles and tighter, thicker skin

※ Strengthened bones

※ Youthful energy production

Seventeen years ago, Daniel Rudman, M.D, of the Medical College of Wisconsin, published a landmark study in the *New England Journal of Medicine*. Dr. Rudman gave human growth hormone to nine men between the ages of sixty-one and eighty-one for only six months. In that short period of time, he was able to show that their physiological age could be reversed approximately 10 percent. These nine men put on muscle and bone, their skin became thicker, and they burned fat in the same way that young men do. All this without any change in alcohol consumption, diet, exercise, or even smoking. These changes were entirely from the growth hormone.

Decreased muscle-to-fat ratio, thinning skin, and decreased bone density are all hallmarks of aging. So what Rudman concluded is that he *reversed the functional age of his patients ten to twenty years simply by restoring their growth-hormone levels to youthful levels.* As hard as it is to believe that result, Rudman's conclusion was based on results he obtained from sound scientific principles that were verified by a placebo-controlled medical study.

Growth hormone is, of course, only one of the hormones that become deficient as people age. How much better his results would have been had he simultaneously replaced other deficient hormones, and placed his patients on an optimum diet, supplement, and lifestyle program.

HORMONAL REPLACEMENT IS THE KEY

Hormones are molecular messengers that operate between the brain and the cells. They control just about every aspect of human function. In addition to energy production, this includes body composition, digestion, healing, immune function, memory and mood, sexual function, skin thickness, strength, and tissue regeneration—everything. When people hear the word hormone, most of them think only of the sex hormones, but there are countless other hormones beside these.

*The major difference between you at age fifty
and you at age twenty-five is hormonal.*

After the reproductive age, say around thirty-five (but in some cases even earlier), the body's production of hormones starts a steady decline. It's a dirty trick that nature plays on people. It's as if to say, "Well, you have reproduced to ensure the perpetuation of the species, so you're not really needed anymore. You can go now."

The question is not *if* you are going to become hormone deficient, rather it is *when*, and *how significant* the deficiencies will be. The rate at which these deficiencies develop determines how fast you will age.

BOTH MEN AND WOMEN

Hormonal deficiencies affect both men and women. Specifically, there are twelve different hormones in women, and eight in men, that become deficient as people age. The symptoms they create include anxiety, bladder disorders, decreased bone mass, decreased muscle mass, decreased sexual drive and function, decreased stamina, declining immune-system function, depression, fatigue, hair loss, increased fat mass, insomnia, reduced equilibrium, reduced mental function, weakness, wrinkles, and above all, decreased energy production.

Hormone deficiencies, especially thyroid hormone deficiencies, can occur even in younger people. Occasionally, I even see them in children. But they usually don't show up until people are in their forties or fifties.

Beside making people age faster, hormone deficiencies also play a major role in the development of most age-related diseases, including Alzheimer's dementia, arthritis, cancer, depression, diabetes, heart disease, osteoporosis, and strokes.

That's the bad news. The good news is that there are now easy, accurate, and reasonably priced ways to test for deficiencies. There are also easy and inexpensive ways to replace sagging levels with bio-identical hormones. By the term bio-identical, I mean hormones that are exact molecular replicas of the hormones they are replacing. With this bio-identical ability, hormone replacement joined the twenty-first century.

While there are definite and significant problems with synthetic hormonal drugs that are still widely used, many long- and short-term studies with both men and women demonstrate the effectiveness of hormone replacement. Not surprisingly, these people live longer and have a much greater quality of life than those not supplemented. The widely publicized problems that have been seen with synthetic hormones have just not been seen with bio-identical hormones. Thanks to bio-identical hormones, hormone deficiencies can now be safely treated as they develop.

HOW ARE HORMONE DEFICIENCIES DETERMINED?

Hormone deficiencies are determined in three different ways. First, a detailed history and physical examination can often diagnose a specific deficiency. After this, laboratory testing can either confirm or negate the condition. And finally, a therapeutic trial can be initiated to see if specific symptoms resolve with proper replacement.

IT's NEVER TOO LATE

Jane had many health problems when she first came to me as a new patient. Although she was only seventy-four-years-old, she had severe chronic lung disease from years of smoking, and could barely walk across the room without help. Her heart was starting to fail and her bones had become quite osteoporotic. Besides her chronic shortness of breath, her main complaint was profound weakness. She took several medications to help her breathe better and was dependent on a supply of oxygen at all times.

Jane had been treated the same as most older people by her medical doctor. According to Jane, he had told her to learn to live with her problems because, "at your age you should be content just to be alive." Sad to say, too many physicians and their patients subscribe to the concept that being weak and feeble are just inevitable features of growing older.

When I first saw Jane, I had to tell her that her lung disease was permanent and could not be repaired. I did add, however, that it was possible to improve her energy production, and hence her overall health, by giving her body back the hormones it had been missing for thirty or more years.

I started Jane on a comprehensive bio-identical hormone-replacement program that included DHEA, estrogens, growth hormone, melatonin, progesterone, testosterone, and thyroid hormones. I also placed her on a high-protein diet with a broad-range program of nutritional supplements. Three short months later, she showed considerable improvement in energy, pain, strength, and sleep. She still needed to take her oxygen bottle wherever she went, but she was finally able to easily ascend the same flight of stairs at home that had previously been extremely difficult for her.

Three years down the road, Jane had made significant across-the-board improvements. Her lung condition did not degenerate. Her bone density was better, as was her heart function. Had it not been for hormone replacement, it is quite possible she would have either been dead or institutionalized. Such improvements, even in someone with as poor health as Jane had, are not unusual. One of the characteristics of bio-identical hormone replacement is that the natural deterioration associated with aging seems to go into reverse gear.

Bless her heart, Jane died peacefully at home eighteen months ago. Her body could no longer subsist on the meager amount of oxygen that her lungs could deliver. While hormonal replacement could never help Jane's serious lung disease, it did give her an extra seven years. Seven **quality** years. During that time she was fully functional right up until twenty days before she left us.

Properly monitoring hormone levels is almost a specialty in itself. There are now newer, more accurate laboratory methods than we've had before. They are much less expensive, and are better able to identify deficiencies.

Currently, the best method for assessing the sex and adrenal hormones is by testing saliva. Blood is much too unreliable for testing these hormones. For thyroid assessment, the most accurate method is Bio-Energy Testing. As you will see, testing thyroid hormones with blood panels is not nearly sensitive enough.

The best way to test for growth-hormone deficiency is through what is called a challenge test. In this test, an amino acid called arginine is given intravenously, and blood levels of growth hormone are checked during and after the infusion.

But when all is said and done, the traditional way of diagnosing a deficiency by talking with and examining the patient is still the best.

WHAT'S SO DIFFERENT ABOUT BIO-IDENTICAL HORMONE REPLACEMENT?

Synthetic hormonal therapy, the conventional way hormones have been replaced, has some serious drawbacks.

Drawback 1

Synthetic hormones are not really hormones at all, they are drugs with hormonelike effects. These commonly prescribed substances are not found in the human body. They are molecularly different from the hormones they are replacing.

Since they are foreign to the body, synthetic hormones not only cannot function properly, they are also treated as toxins by the liver. According to several studies on the use of these synthetic hormones, side effects prompt up to 30 percent of all the people placed on these so-called wonders to stop using them within twelve months.

All this begs the question, "If I am deficient in a particular hormone, why isn't the deficiency treated with that exact hormone?" Unfortunately, the reason has nothing to do with good medicine, or even common sense. The answer lies in the economic fact that molecules, such as hormones, that occur naturally in the body are not patentable. This means, therefore, they are not profitable for the drug companies to sell.

The good news, however, is that bio-identical hormone therapy—using hormones that are molecularly identical to the hormones they are replacing—is now readily available. And it is being used by many doctors all over the world.

Drawback 2

The conventional approach completely ignores the fact that hormones work together as a team. Although each individual hormone has its own specific actions, it also requires other hormones to be present in order to function properly. *Since any given hormone can enhance the action of one hormone while suppressing another, too much or too little of one hormone can create an imbalance in other hormones.*

The system of hormonal checks and balances is the way the body regulates itself. If a person is deficient in two hormones, she or he should replace both hormones. If deficient in seven hormones, for optimum results all seven should be replaced. Conventional replacement strategy ignores these important interrelationships.

Drawback 3

The conventional approach tends to embrace a one-size-fits-all mentality. Individual hormone deficiencies vary greatly. Therefore, the correct dose for one person with a particular hormone deficiency may be very different from another person. *In the conventional approach, it is quite common for people to take either too much or too little of a hormone.* The only reliable way to discover these differences is to monitor each person's response with a series of hormone tests and clinical evaluations, both before and during replacement therapy.

MY THREE GOLDEN RULES

To avoid these problems, I follow three golden rules in regard to hormone replacement that have worked well for me over the years.

Golden Rule 1

I use only bio-identical hormones—the exact same hormones that occur naturally in the human body. It has never made any sense to me to replace the human hormone estradiol with the horse hormones that comprise Premarin, the most commonly prescribed estrogen replacement for women.

Similarly, since natural progesterone is available, and is identical to the body's own progesterone, why use a patented substitute drug like Provera? But this is what most physicians use. Foreign substances, such as Provera, set off immune responses in the body that frequently cause complications. These complications simply don't occur when bio-identical hormones are used.

Golden Rule 2

Using comprehensive laboratory hormonal assessment, I replace all hormone deficiencies present, not just the ones that give the effect I'm looking for. This helps maintain a youthful balance of hormones, and it allows me to use much lower individual hormone doses and still get the same effects.

Golden Rule 3

I individualize all doses, and prescribe just enough, not too much, of each hormone. One size definitely does not fit all. Even twins may have widely divergent levels of hormones. The best dose of any hormone is the lowest one that gets the job done.

CUSTOMIZING DOSAGES

Because of the need for individual dosing, standardized capsules or creams are never used in bio-identical replacement. All bio-identical hormone-replacement capsules and creams are made up individually for each person.

The process of making a customized capsule or cream for a particular person is called compounding. These customized medications can be obtained from one of the many compounding pharmacies located through-

HOW BIO-IDENTICAL HORMONES ARE MADE

Bio-identical hormones are made in laboratories from precursor molecules that are naturally produced in a plant called wild yam. These precurser molecules are very similar in construction to the estrogen hormones, testosterone, and progesterone. A few quick bio-chemical reactions, and poof, the chemist can change the precursor molecules into the same identical homone molecules that are found in the body. Compounding pharmacists then buy these hormones from the chemical suppliers, and use them to create pills, capsules, suppositories, and creams for human use.

out the country. Compounding pharmacies specialize in making hormone prescriptions, and other preparations, directly from raw materials and according to the exact recommendations of your doctor. Because of this, the compounding pharmacist is able to customize the exact ratio of hormones that your particular body needs. At regular, non-compounding pharmacies, the only bio-identical hormones you can get are the standard one-size-fits-all dosages supplied by drug manufacturers.

IS IT SAFE *NOT* TO REPLACE HORMONAL DEFICIENCIES?

The most frequent question I hear from my patients regarding bio-identical hormone replacement is the obvious one: Is it safe? I believe it is among the safest of all medical treatments. But, to be honest, although I have been safely prescribing bio-identical hormones for over fifteen years now, there are still no published studies that have examined this question. Moreover, I tell my patients that the most significant danger regarding bio-identical hormonal replacement is *not* doing it.

And so I ask another question: Is it safe *not* to replace hormones when there is a deficiency? Although the scientific and clinical data on this issue can be criticized from all sides, the evidence strongly suggests that denying a person bio-identical hormonal replacement is dangerous. It is just as dangerous as denying a person with high blood pressure appropriate treatment.

For example, in every long-term human study that has looked at estrogen-replacement therapy, those on estrogen replacement lived longer, had a lower incidence of disease, and had a higher quality of life than comparison groups who did not take the hormone.

According to one published study of 8881 post-menopausal women, *"Current users with more than 15 years of estrogen use had a 40-percent reduction in their overall mortality."* That's a lot. The users also had reduced mortality from cancer.

The same kind of data is available for men as well. Several studies evaluating older men on testosterone replacement therapy have found no side effects or dangers of any consequence. Many doctors are still concerned about what might happen to the prostate of men on testosterone-replacement therapy, but so far no problems have been encountered. What's more, research has shown a positive impact on cholesterol that reduces the risk of death from cardiovascular disease.

These gratifying results occurred in spite of the fact that the research was done with synthetic hormone drugs. I can only wonder how much better the results would have been had the hormones been bio-identical.

Several short-term human studies have demonstrated that replacement with bio-identical hormones generates a host of significant rejuvenating effects. Animal studies have verified such results.

THE PLAYERS

There are basically two different categories of hormones—the catabolic hormones and the anabolic hormones. Both are major players in total energy production.

Catabolic hormones receive this designation because they directly stimulate the mitochondria to produce more energy. The process is called catabolism. The thyroid hormones and the adrenal hormones, cortisol and adrenalin, are the most potent catabolic hormones.

The anabolic hormones increase energy production in a different way. They don't directly stimulate the mitochondria to go to work. Instead, by stimulating protein synthesis, organ repair, and other cellular processes, they use up the energy that the mitochondria produce. By using up energy, they then create a requirement for more energy. This is critical to mitochondrial function because one thing about mitochondria is that they are not able to produce energy unless there is an energy demand. The anabolic hormones supply this demand.

The most important anabolic hormones are DHEA, estrogen, growth hormone, melatonin progesterone, and testosterone. Properly replacing both anabolic and catabolic hormones increases longevity and decreases disease by keeping energy production at more youthful levels.

ABOUT ESTROGENS

Estrogen is not one, but three hormones that have played a dominant role in the medical research and application of hormone replacement therapy. For that reason, I'll be using the plural—estrogens.

In most people's minds, the word hormone is synonymous with estrogens, and the reason is quite simple. The estrogens are the most powerful hormones in the female body—almost every cell membrane has receptor sites (areas of activity) specific for estrogens.

These compounds affect everything from the way a woman thinks to the way she looks. They exert a profound influence on the arteries, bladder, bones, brain, fat cells, liver, soft tissues of the joints and muscles, thyroid gland, and cellular metabolism in general.

Estrogens decrease the clotting tendency of the blood, keep the blood thin, and cause a marked improvement in the HDL/LDL cholesterol ratio—they are the reason that heart attacks and strokes occur much less frequently in women. They are also extremely powerful antioxidants, and in this way retard the aging process in general.

Since estrogens stimulate the synthesis of choline acetyl-transferase, an important brain enzyme that is lacking in Alzheimer's disease, a deficiency of estrogens is regarded as a primary cause of this disease in women. Even without the extreme of outright Alzheimer's disease, a deficiency in estrogens can result in mood swings, forgetfulness, and difficulty in concentration.

The wrinkles that begin to develop after menopause are primarily secondary to a deficiency in estrogens. That's because these hormones enhance the production of collagen, and keep the skin thick and hydrated.

Estrogens also prevent the facial hair growth that is common after menopause. A deficiency of estrogen not only paves the way for osteoporosis, but is also behind many of the other diseases associated with aging women. According to Uzzi Reiss, MD, who authored an excellent book, *Natural Hormone Balance for Women*, women with estrogen deficiency often experience a decreased sense of *womaness*, and report a diminished self-image, sensuality, and sexuality.

HALF THE DEATH RATE

One of the most famous studies on the benefits of estrogens came out of the Oakland Kaiser Permanente Medical Care Program in 1996. The study monitored 232 women who for years had been taking estradiol, the most potent estrogen compound. These women were compared with a control group of other women who did not take any hormones. The results showed that women taking the estradiol had nearly half the overall death rate of those who didn't. Deaths from cancer were essentially the same in both groups.

Despite this study and others like it, estrogens replacement therapy (ERT) has received a rash of criticism it doesn't deserve. The criticism stems mostly from the fact that ERT, as it is conventionally administered, uses synthetic hormones. *In my practice, I routinely recommend ERT to my women patients, but never conventional ERT.* It's been proven to be too dangerous. Conventional ERT has been found to increase the risk of breast cancer, heart attacks, and strokes. This risk has not been seen when using bio-identical hormones.

I use only bio-identical hormones in my practice, and there is no evidence they have the same effect. Why? Because the differences between these two approaches—bio-identical and conventional—are huge. For starters, conventional replacement therapy isn't replacement therapy at all. It's drug therapy.

The definition of replacement therapy implies that a molecule found deficient in the human body is replaced by the identical molecule. But conventional ERT does not follow this maxim. Instead, it uses patented drugs, such as Premarin. The drug Premarin does not contain bio-identical estrogens. It contains horse estrogens made from the urine of pregnant mares.

As my good friend Jonathan Wright, M.D., a pioneer in the science of bio-identical hormonal replacement, has been saying for years, *"Premarin is replacement therapy for horses, but it is drug therapy for humans."* No wonder Premarin and other synthetic estrogens cause problems in humans. They don't belong in the human body.

A reasonable person may ask, "If human estrogens are available, why are physicians prescribing synthetic estrogens?" As I explained earlier, the answer has nothing to do with good medicine. The reason is not medical, it's economic. It stems from the fact that the law does not allow the drug companies to patent a *naturally occurring substance.* And without a patent on a medication, there is no way for a drug company to make a decent profit from it. The pharmaceutical industry is a multi-billion dollar, for-profit corporate industry. There's nothing wrong with that. It's just that, like any other industry, it's primary interest is the bottom line. And since the FDA demands very extensive tests and clinical investigations before any pharmaceutical treatment can be approved, it does not make good business sense to market a non-patentable substance. The end result of this situation is that you receive a patentable combination containing horse estrogens or other synthetics instead of the real thing.

IT'S A BALANCING ACT

Another problem with conventional prescriptions of estrogens relates to lack of balance. There are three estrogen compounds in the body—estradiol, estrone, and estriol. Estradiol is the most powerful, and in the body, estrone and estriol interact with estradiol and keep it in check. This is the body's intelligence at work. It's a balancing act. And balance is critical to hormones because they have such major effects in the body. That is why nature put three estrogens in the body, not just one.

To replace an estradiol deficiency with estradiol, but neglect to replace an estriol or estrone deficiency doesn't make good sense. Moreover, it can be dangerous.

The pharmaceutical companies have patented a delivery system called the estradiol patch to enhance the introduction of the compound into the body. There has been much advertising hoopla about this new form of ERT because they are actually using the bio-identical form of estradiol. The problem with the estradiol patch, however, is that it's not balanced with estrone and estriol.

When I give ERT to my patients, I prescribe all three compounds in a balanced formula. They are natural and bio-identical to what a woman normally has in her body. I always individualize the dose for each woman based on testing and retesting her hormonal status.

CREAMS VERSUS PILLS

Another important consideration concerning natural ERT is how the estrogens are administered. Estrogen taken in pill or capsule form upsets the balance of other hormones, such as the growth hormone IGF-1, testosterone, and the thyroid hormones.

Since oral estrogen goes immediately to the liver after it is absorbed, very high concentrations build up in the liver. This high level of estrogen has several effects on the way the liver regulates hormones. For example, the growth hormone IGF-1 is made in the liver, and high concentrations of estrogen cause the liver to make less IGF-1, thus creating a growth-hormone deficiency.

The next problem with oral estrogen has to do with a hormone-carrying protein called sex-hormone-binding globulin (SHBG). SHBG is a carrier protein that is formed in the liver. It binds to both estradiol and testosterone. The good news is that SHBG preserves healthy levels of estradiol and testosterone because as long as they are bound to SHBG they will not be lost in the urine. The bad news is that when hormones are bound to SHBG, they cannot exert their hormonal effects. It's as if they weren't there as far as the body is concerned.

So when too much SHBG is present, the hormones are excessively bound up and can't work. And that's the problem with oral estrogen. Because so much of it is concentrated in the liver, the liver responds by making too much SHBG. The excess SHBG binds up so much testosterone that the body experiences a lack of testosterone activity.

As one study points out, testosterone is not only an important hormone for sexual functioning, but it is also important for muscle maintenance. The researchers looked at forty-six postmenopausal women who were taking oral estrogen and compared them to women not taking any hormones. The SHBG levels of the women on the oral estrogen were so high that their testosterone levels were excessively bound up. This caused them to have a significant reduction in their muscle mass.

Oral estrogen has a similar effect on the thyroid hormones. It causes the liver to make too much thyroid-hormone-binding globulin. This globulin binds up thyroid hormones and results in low thyroid function.

For all these reasons, I much prefer to use topical creams over estrogen capsules and pills. The creams do not affect IGF-1 production or cause any increase in SHBG because they pass through the skin rather than the liver.

ABOUT PROGESTERONE

Progesterone is a critical hormone in the reproductive cycle. After a woman ovulates, she produces progesterone in the ovaries to prepare the uterus for conception and the development of the fertilized egg.

But progesterone plays many other important and protective roles in a woman's body.

☀ It contributes to a healthier LDL/HDL cholesterol ratio.

☀ It enhances the activity of the thyroid hormone on energy production.

☀ It has a calming effect on mood.

☀ It helps balance the estrogens.

☀ It helps prevent abnormal blood clotting.

☀ It helps stabilize blood sugar.

☀ It improves the sex drive.

☀ It is a natural diuretic, and as such decreases edema and subsequent cellulite formation.

☀ It is a powerful antioxidant.

☀ It prevents breast and uterine cancer.

☀ It stimulates formation of new bone tissue. The estrogens decrease bone loss. Progesterone promotes new bone growth.

☀ It supports healthy sleep.

The list could go on, but it's enough to show you what an extremely important hormone this is. Unfortunately, however, progesterone levels generally start to decline when a woman reaches her mid-thirties. By the time a woman reaches the age of forty-five, the decline accelerates so fast that it quickly becomes deficient. Because of all the remarkable benefits listed above, women in this category should consider replacing deficient progesterone levels as soon as they occur.

ESTROGEN DOMINANCE

Estrogen and progesterone oppose each other. Whatever one does, the other un-does. This is very common in the body. One hormone does one thing, and another does the opposite—this is the way the body can regulate itself. A deficiency of progesterone is equivalent to an excess of estrogen. When either the progesterone levels decline or the estrogen levels increase, the condition is referred to as estrogen dominance.

Estrogen dominance causes havoc in a woman's body. Breast and uterine cancer, cellulite, endometriosis, fibrocystic breast disease, PMS, water retention, and weight gain are all side effects of estrogen dominance. And it is as big a problem with young women as it is with the older set.

The most common manifestation of estrogen dominance is PMS, with its symptoms of anxiety, breast swelling, depression, insomnia, irritability, loss of libido, pelvic pain, and water retention. This is low progesterone at work, and it can be corrected by either lowering estrogen levels and/or replacing low progesterone levels. But what causes estrogen dominance in the first place?

Estrogen dominance initially stems from a combination of decreased liver function and an excessive environmental exposure to *xenoestrogens*. Xenoestrogens is a term referring to synthetic chemicals that can act like human estrogens. These compounds are used everywhere—in fungicides, sunscreens, herbicides, pesticides, solvents, paper, and plastics. You can't escape them.

Over the years, xenoestrogens have thoroughly infiltrated the food chain. Every time you eat, you're getting a barrage of these estrogenlike compounds. The highest exposures come from beef and chicken because they are routinely dosed up with estrogens to increase their weight and fat content. You can buy hormone-free meats, but you have to look for them in the supermarket. Please do that.

Make no mistake about it, xenoestrogens are a real problem. They are believed to contribute to the rise in sterility commonly seen in young people. Many researchers feel they are also behind the growing incidence of premature secondary sex characteristics developing in children.

Xenoestrogens, Suppressed Ovulation, and Estrogen Dominance

Ovulation occurs about ten days after the menstrual period begins. This triggers the production of progesterone. As xenoestrogens build up in the body, however, they can suppress normal ovulation, causing progesterone production to dramatically decrease. The result: Estrogen dominance.

Suppressed Ovulation—More Common Than Is Realized

Traditionally, doctors have always thought that as long as a woman was menstruating, she must be ovulating. It was thought that suppressed ovulation occurred only rarely in regularly menstruating women. But recent research shows it is much more common than previously realized, and can easily occur in a menstruating woman.

Birth control pills also suppress ovulation, and inasmuch as they contain strong synthetic estrogen compounds, they can drastically increase estrogen dominance.

As women approach their mid-forties, suppressed ovulation becomes even more commonplace. The estrogen dominance that ensues causes cellulite and weight gain around the hips, and increases the risk of breast and uterine cancer.

One solution to this would be for everyone to avoid the *–cides* (pesticides, fungicides, and herbicides), and eat only hormone-free beef and chicken. An additional measure should also include not storing foods in soft plastic wraps. Soft plastics are loaded with xenoestrogens, which can easily be absorbed from the plastic into the food wrapped in the plastic. But this is not a perfect world, and the chances of avoiding all exposure to xenoestrogens is slim.

Another, very accessible and powerful strategy to combat the buildup of xenoestrogens is to take the nutrients in QuickStart. This particular combination promotes detoxification, and gives significant nutritional support to the liver. It is the liver that is ultimately responsible for removing the xenoestrogens you have been exposed to from your system, and it needs all the help you can give it. Along with these nutrients, regular exercise and a high-fiber diet will help the clean-up process.

BUT MY DOCTOR SAYS

Doctors often tell their patients that a woman who has had a hysterectomy doesn't need progesterone replacement. I guess if a woman were simply a large uterus with legs, they would have a point. But the truth is, such a statement disregards the fact that every cell in a woman's body has progesterone-receptor sites. Bones have receptors. So does the brain. So do the breasts, and the liver, the bladder, and the skin—every cell. Progesterone is just as important to these cells as it is to the uterus.

A woman needs progesterone whether or not she has a uterus. Furthermore, this fact is greatly exaggerated in the presence of estrogen dominance because estrogen opposes progesterone. When all those cells have decreased levels of progesterone activating their receptors, it causes a whole host of problems that so many otherwise normal healthy women often experience. Problems such as anxiety, cellulite, endometriosis, fatigue, fibrocystic breasts, gallstones, insomnia, irritability, menstrual pain, migraines, panic disorder, PMS, uterine fibroids, water retention, and weight gain. Give these women progesterone and a wonderful thing happens. Most of the time these problems all go away like magic.

PROVERA IS NOT PROGESTERONE

One more comment about progesterone. More specifically about Provera, a drug masquerading as progesterone. Even though it is not progesterone, Provera is routinely prescribed by doctors as a progesterone replacement. Provera is a drug, not a hormone. If it were a hormone, it would not be patentable, and would not be nearly as profitable for drug companies to manufacture. But since it is a drug, it *is* patentable, and, as such, it has been heavily promoted for years as a viable substitute for the real thing.

Make no mistake about it, though—it may be a pharmaceutical bestseller, but it is a nightmare for the human body. If there is some legitimate use for this drug, I don't know what it is. Like any physician, I appreciate that some of the drugs developed by the pharmaceutical industry have saved many lives. But Provera is not one of them. It should be taken off the market because it is one of the worst drugs currently available.

If you take a look at the Physicans' Desk Reference (PDR), and check out the common side effects of this drug, you would wonder why anyone would prescribe it. The list reads like a who's who of symptoms: acne, birth defects, blood clots, breast cancer, breast tenderness, dementia, depression, diabetes, facial hair growth, fatigue, fluid retention, head hair loss, heart disease, pulmonary embolism, rashes, strokes, and weight gain.

Bio-identical progesterone has none of these problems. So why would anyone want to take this drug, or any other drug in this class of progesterone substitutes called progestins, when real, natural progesterone is readily available?

The answer is, they take the drug because that's what their doctors prescribe. Hard as it is to believe, I have talked with many doctors who don't even know that Provera is not progesterone. Other doctors are just unaware of the bio-identical option. Still others mistakenly believe that bio-identical progesterone doesn't work because their drug retailers are not pushing it. And many of their patients, particularly those not up on the latest in medicine, don't know about it.

I find that a topical progesterone cream works best for the majority of my women patients. This is because progesterone is notoriously poor at being absorbed when taken orally. There are some excellent bio-identical progesterone creams available over the counter. If you decide to use one of these creams, be sure to find a physician who is familiar with their use. Also be sure to check your salivary progesterone levels after you are on it a few weeks just to be sure you are taking the correct dose. Blood levels of progesterone won't do. Only a salivary specimen can follow this hormone.

THYROID HORMONES—THE MASTER HORMONES

The thyroid gland has the primary responsibility for stimulating your mitochondria to produce energy. *All* aspects of energy production are dependent on the actions of the thyroid hormones. Without an adequate amount of the two thyroid hormones, T_3 and T_4, your cells would cease working and you would die. It's no wonder then that the symptoms associated with a malfunctioning thyroid read like a litany of what can go wrong in the human body.

More than half the American men and women older than forty experience *three or more* symptoms related to a thyroid hormone deficiency, a condition referred to as hypothyroidism. And past the age of fifty, it is fairly uncommon to have an optimally functioning thyroid.

The thyroid gland, wrapped around the front of your windpipe just below the Adam's apple, produces these master hormones. They are called master hormones for a very simple reason: *All the other hormones are dependent on them for their own optimal functioning.* Even if you have optimal levels of other hormones, they will not work properly if you are deficient in your levels of T_3 and T_4.

BRODA BARNES, M.D.—MASTER CLINICIAN

Years ago, when I first began to study alternative medical treatments, I read an important book on the unrecognized prevalence of hypothyroidism, and the importance of thyroid replacement. The book was written in 1976 by Broda Barnes, M.D. Dr. Barnes was a veteran physician who went way back to the days when medicine was practiced as a clinical art, instead of just a recitation of laboratory tests. He felt the best way to determine the presence of a thyroid deficiency was to monitor the body temperature using a basal thermometer.

It is a simple enough procedure, so I began having my patients take their underarm temperature when they awoke in the morning. It didn't take long before I realized that probably no more than 5 percent of my patients had a normal reading. If Barnes was correct, the great majority of my patients needed thyroid replacement. This was despite the fact that almost all of them tested normal for thyroid using standard laboratory tests.

I was confused. And to make matters even more confusing, Barnes said the correct thyroid dose was one that restored temperatures to an optimum level. *In order to accomplish this though, I would have to give many of my patients thyroid doses that were much higher than what was considered by some to be the maximum output of an adult thyroid.*

But I decided to try the Barnes approach anyway. It was, after all, based on his thirty-five years of clinical experience with thousands of patients. Soon, *my* patients started telling me the same things Barnes's patients had reported to him—that they had never felt so good in all their lives. Many of their long-standing and unresolved symptoms had simply vanished.

Barnes, the old master clinician, had apparently discovered something very profound that was completely perplexing to me. How was it possible that almost everyone I tested using the temperature test was found to have low thyroid function? How could so many patients do so well on thyroid doses that most experts would regard as excessive? It wasn't until almost twenty years later, when I began using Bio-Energy Testing, that I was finally able to answer these questions.

WHY DOES ALMOST EVERYONE NEED THYROID?

No one really knows exactly why the decline in thyroid function is so common. Perhaps it is simply the effect of aging. The levels of all the other hormones decrease with age, so why shouldn't the thyroid hormones? There are few things more certain than a decline in the metabolic rate associated with aging. And since thyroid hormones control the metabolic rate, it seems very probable that decreased thyroid function is just one of the things that happens as people get older.

But thyroid-hormone decline can also occur from excessive fluoride supplementation, excessive bromine intake, selenium, iodine, and zinc deficiency, silver dental fillings (they contain mercury that is highly toxic to the thyroid gland), and chiropractic, dental, and medical x-rays. These are commonplace factors, and all probably play roles behind an underfunctioning thyroid.

The female hormone estrogen interferes with thyroid hormone function. Women always have a lower metabolic rate than men because of this effect of estrogen. And estrogen dominance decreases thyroid function even more. Paradoxically, a thyroid decline also results in lack of ovulation in women, which is a primary cause of estrogen dominance.

WHY DO PEOPLE SOMETIMES NEED
EXCESSIVE THYROID DOSES?

The answers lie beyond the thyroid itself—with the hypothalamus, a center within the brain, and with the body's good friend, the liver.

The hypothalamus is the hormone thermostat for the body, and it is very sensitive to the body's need for thyroid hormones. When it senses that the body's metabolic rate is too slow, it sends a signal to the pituitary gland to release thyroid stimulating hormone (TSH). TSH then goes to the thyroid and stimulates it to make T_4, an inactive form of the thyroid hormone (by inactive, I mean that T_4 is not able to stimulate energy production). T_4 then circulates through the bloodstream to the liver where it is converted into T_3, the active thyroid hormone. T_3 is responsible for stimulating the cells to increase their energy production, so they can function properly.

The liver converts T_4 to T_3 on a demand basis. When there is a greater need for a stepped-up metabolism, for example to support increased activity, such as exercise, the liver responds by making more T_3. As more T_3 is made, it exerts what is known as a negative feedback to the hypothalamus, which turns down the production of TSH. This causes the thyroid to decrease its production of T_4, which, in turn, prevents too much T_3 from being produced and burning out the mitochondria. This elaborate and complex control mechanism is called the thyroid axis (see figure at right).

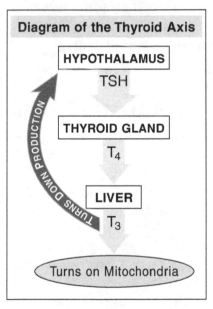

I believe the reason some of my patients thrive on high doses of thyroid is that there is a breakdown in one or more aspects of this axis. In many cases, the problem may be a sluggish liver. In that case, a revitalization of the liver will allow lower thyroid doses to be just as effective. In other cases, the problem may lie in the hypothalamus.

BIO-ENERGY TESTING TO THE RESCUE

Many people are relegated to permanent misery simply because they have what is described in the medical literature as sub-clinical hypothyroidism.

This means people, such as my patient Loretta, who have low thyroid function in the face of lab results that fall within the statistical normal range. A 1983 study published in *Postgraduate Medicine* and titled, "How to detect hypothyroidism when screening tests are normal," covered this issue.

In the study, sixty-five women, such as Loretta, were examined because of their many symptoms suggestive of hypothyroidism. In all cases, the blood tests were within normal range. Using a sophisticated stimulation challenge test, the researchers demonstrated that forty-seven of the women, 72 percent, did in fact have hypothyroidism despite the normal tests. It's no surprise that when they were treated with thyroid hormone, they improved.

Other studies have revealed that in any given age group somewhere between 5–15 percent of the population has laboratory-detectable subclinical hypothyroidism. One of the great advantages of Bio-Energy Testing is that since it measures metabolic rate, it is the most sensitive way to determine the presence of low-thyroid function even when subclinical hypothyroidism is present.

LORETTA'S PROBLEM SOLVED AND RE-SOLVED

Loretta is one of many people I have treated over the years who dramatically demonstrates the heavy, unreliable dependence many physicians have on thyroid blood testing.

Loretta was fifty-two-years-old and healthy, according to her previous physician. This, despite the fact she had been complaining of dry skin, fatigue, intolerance for cold, lack of energy, and weight gain, for eight years. She also had an increasing cholesterol level.

Loretta had done her homework. She knew that her symptoms and her elevated cholesterol are often related to a low thyroid. Over the years, she repeatedly asked her doctor to give her a trial dose of thyroid hormone. Her doctor, however, was wedded to the thyroid blood tests, and refused to do so because her results had always been in the normal range.

Finally, she came to my clinic because she had read an article I wrote regarding the inaccuracy of thyroid blood testing. Using Bio-Energy Testing, I checked her M-Factor. A decreased M-Factor indicates hypothyroidism (low-thyroid function). I was not at all surprised to find she was running at about 60 percent of optimum. Since she had many of the symptoms of hypothyroidism, I started her on a trial of thyroid-hormone replacement.

Loretta lived out of town, and called me in about four weeks to say elatedly, "I feel like I've been given a second chance at life." Her symptoms were gone, and her cholesterol readings were much improved.

TESTOSTERONE

Testosterone is considered the male sex hormone. But it doesn't belong exclusively to men. Women's bodies also make a small, but important, amount that greatly contributes to their health. In both women and men, a testosterone deficiency leads to apathy, depression, a diminished or lost sex drive, fat gain, joint aches and pains, loss of exercise endurance, and osteoporosis. There is almost always a deficiency in women who have had a hysterectomy.

But back to the men. Unlike women, who have been studied for sex-hormone deficiency for decades, testosterone deficiencies in men have largely been ignored in this country. Women experience a rapid decline of sex hormones, but the loss of testosterone in men is often quite slow, taking effect very gradually over ten to fifteen years. And because it occurs

---

A couple of years went by before I heard from her again. She had sprained her ankle a few months before and had seen her regular doctor for treatment. When he learned she had been taking thyroid replacement, he became quite upset, insisting that all her tests failed to show the need for the hormone.

Loretta explained the results of her testing, but like many physicians he was unfamiliar with Bio-Energy Testing. He took some blood tests again, and even though the results were still in the normal range, he insisted that she discontinue the thyroid hormones. He never explained why her blood test results were within normal limits both **on** and **off** thyroid replacement. Of course the reason is that they are just not that accurate.

Because of his insistence, she stopped taking the thyroid hormones. Predictably, within two weeks, she began to notice a return of her symptoms. When she saw her doctor two months later, she was back to feeling as bad as ever. In spite of this rather obvious clinical example of thyroid-hormone deficiency, her physician continued to maintain she didn't need any replacement therapy because the "blood tests are all normal." He appeared happier with a miserable patient who had normal tests than with a well patient who **also** had normal lab tests.

It may seem strange, but some physicians are more devoted to laboratory results than they are to how their patients are feeling. Needless to say, Loretta had had enough. She was smart enough to listen to her body, so she called my clinic. I restarted her on the hormone replacement she so obviously needed, and she immediately began to regain her health.

---

so slowly, men seldom fully realize the nature of what has happened to them.

Another reason why men just haven't gotten equal treatment is related to the male ego, and the "nothing-is-wrong" mentality. I routinely see this attitude among my patients who are men. Sometimes it is almost comical. Here's a typical example of an interview in my office with a man in his 50s or 60s.

Me: "So how's your sex life?"

Him: "Not a problem."

Me: "OK, how about your memory?"

Him: "Not a problem."

Me: "Great. How about your moods?"

Him: "Seem fine."

Me: "And how's your strength and stamina?"

Him: "No complaints there either, Doc."

Me: "OK. Now I want you to compare how all these things are to how they were ten or fifteen years ago."

He thinks for a few moments.

"Of course, I'm not the man I used to be," he admits. "Those were the days. Nothing could get me down. I could have sex all the time, stay out all night long, and get up in the morning and . . ."

Often, it's only when men honestly compare their current level of function to their peak years that they realize there has been a definite decline.

Grumpy Old Men

Few things in medicine are as rewarding to me as replacing a depleted man's testosterone. Few things seem to be as rewarding to the man's wife as well.

I vividly remember the morning I walked into the clinic and saw a gorgeous arrangement of roses on the counter. Being a big lover of flowers, I immediately asked, "Well, who did what to get those?" The answer from the staff was, "That's what we'd like to know. They're for you."

The card was from one of my women patients and read as follows:

> *"Roses are red,*
> *Violets are blue,*
> *My husband's a stud,*
> *All thanks to you!"*

And it wasn't just his renewed interest in sex, a result of testosterone replacement, that had this lady so pleased. It was also his remarkable improvement in mood.

Testosterone has a marked uplifting effect on the mood of both men and women. The positive enthusiasm, passion, and risk-taking so characteristic of men is mediated by testosterone. As men age and their testosterone levels decrease, they tend to become grumpy, irritable, apathetic, and listless.

Tiberius Reiter, M.D., first reported the benefits of testosterone replacement for men back in the early 1960s. After twelve years, and 240 patients who complained of premature aging, he described the following results: "Men who were stooped, slow moving, slow thinking, and considering retirement like old men, came back for a check-up at two months looking quite different. They walk well, hold themselves erect, and talk and act like very young fifty-year-olds instead of very old sixty-year-olds. There is even a change in the voice, manner, and handshake."

Testosterone and Your Heart

Testosterone and the heart is a connection most doctors miss. The fact is, testosterone exerts marked protective and therapeutic effects on the heart. This shouldn't seem too strange because the heart is a muscle, after all, and testosterone exerts a powerful effect on muscle function. The benefit is particularly significant for men who have diabetes, but it also applies to all men with heart disease.

Testosterone deficiency causes an undesirable decrease in the HDL/LDL cholesterol ratio which is associated with atherosclerosis. In addition, it contributes to coronary artery blockage, elevated blood pressure, elevated triglycerides, an increased tendency for blood clotting, and insulin resistance.

Testosterone replacement reverses these negative developments. People report improvements on many fronts, including blood clotting, cardiac function, chest pain, cholesterol profiles, glucose control, treadmill testing, and weight management. Men (and women) with heart disease should definitely explore testosterone-replacement therapy.

Testosterone and Your Prostate

Fearing it will aggravate the prostate, many doctors shy away from testosterone replacement. This fear persists despite the reality that both prostate cancer and prostate enlargement only develop in older men with lower testosterone levels.

I carefully monitor the prostate status of my patients on testosterone replacement, just as I routinely do with all the men I treat who are older than fifty. With proper testosterone replacement therapy, the only effect I usually see on the prostate is *improvement*. PSA tests improve. Bladder function improves. I have never seen the opposite occur. Perhaps this is because I also carefully monitor the estrogen level. Yes, men have some estrogen, just as women have some testosterone. And, as men age and their testosterone levels go down, their estrogen levels go up. These elevated estrogen levels are what causes a swollen prostate (called benign prostatic hypertrophy—BPH) so common to men as they get older.

Testosterone replacement can stimulate an increase in estrogen levels in men. When this unpleasant complication occurs, it can be usually be treated by optimizing liver function, and taking an extract of the passionflower plant. This plant has the ability to effectively block the conversion of testosterone to estrogen.

Another important concept regarding testosterone conversion to estrogen in men has to do with how the testosterone is administered. While testosterone injections are notorious for causing this problem, testosterone creams and implants are much less likely to have this effect. When these steps are taken, I have yet to see a complication from testosterone replacement.

In his 1998 book, *Maximizing Manhood*, British physician Malcolm Carruthers describes his experience treating more than a thousand men with testosterone replacement. He writes that after a half-century of testosterone treatment for men with low testosterone levels, there is no evidence of any associated rise in prostate cancer or benign prostatic hypertrophy.

Testosterone replacement does not cause prostate cancer. However, *men who have prostate cancer* need to know that testosterone replacement will induce the cancer to grow at an accelerated rate. With this in mind, I do not administer testosterone to any of my patients with a history of prostate cancer.

But many men have prostate cancer that is so small they don't know they have it. So just in case, for the first year that I give testosterone replacement to any man, I check his PSA test every three months. If he has an undiagnosed prostate cancer, its presence will become apparent, because we will see the PSA steadily climb. I have had a few patients like this. In each case, I was glad to have administered the testosterone because, if I hadn't, the cancer would not have been discovered as early as it was.

THE AMAZING HUMAN GROWTH HORMONE

The longer I use human growth hormone (hGH) replacement, the more amazed I am. More than any other hormone, hGH has the most stunning and wide-ranging anti-aging properties. It significantly influences all aspects of aging, including the production of other hormones.

According to Daniel Rudman, M.D., "The overall deterioration of the body that comes with growing old is not inevitable . . . We now realize that some aspects of it can be prevented or reversed."

In a 2000 article published in *Hormone Research*, the author concludes that life without growth hormone is poor in quality and quantity. He further makes the point that typical growth-hormone levels of men in their sixties are "indistinguishable" from people with documented diseases of the pituitary gland.

The only limitation to the use of growth hormone has been the cost factor. Just ten years ago, a month's supply of hGH would cost you $10,000. Thanks to recombinant DNA technology, and the fact that the growth-hormone patents have run out, hGH can now be produced at a much more reasonable price. Today, a month's supply costs about $200.

Human growth hormone is named after the growth spurts synonymous with the teenage years. An enormous increase of hGH sparks this high-growth period. During this time of life, hGH blood levels can soar to as much as 2,000 mcg/L per day.

What goes up, must come down, so after the sharp rise during the growth spurt, there is a falloff. The average amount of hGH produced at age twenty is about 600 mcg/L. At thirty, about 400 mcg/L, and by forty, the level is down to 250 mcg/L. From here, it tends to decrease very slow-ly over the next forty years to a lowly average of 25 mcg/L per day.

The elevated levels seen in the teenage years drive growth. The lower levels in adulthood maintain that growth.

As you grow older, when your hGH levels start sagging below 200 mcg/L, your body will also begin to sag—and shrink as well. Ever so slowly. That's right. Your brain, heart, liver, lungs, and all the rest, actually reduce in size.

This downsizing is referred to as atrophy. You see it most noticeably as sagging muscles and skin. And you feel it most noticeably in the form of diminished functioning.

☀ As the bones atrophy, you develop osteoporosis and become shorter.

☀ As the brain shrinks, you are not able to think as quickly and as clear-ly as you once could.

☀ As the heart atrophies, you won't have the stamina and endurance you had.

☀ As the hormone-producing glands atrophy, you will have lower and lower levels of hormones.

☀ As the immune system atrophies, your resistance will diminish and you will be more likely to develop infectious illnesses and cancer.

☀ As your muscles atrophy, you will start to lose your strength and your physique.

☀ As your skin atrophies, you will develop wrinkles.

Replacing deficient levels of growth hormone can slow down all those losses and, in many cases, even reverse the process, as the following *Documented Benefits of hGH Therapy* indicate.

DOCUMENTED BENEFITS OF HGH THERAPY

An 8.8 percent increase in muscle mass in six months without exercise

A 14.4 percent loss of fat mass in six months without dieting

- ❑ Enhanced sexual performance
- ❑ Faster healing
- ❑ Higher energy levels
- ❑ Improved brain function
- ❑ Improved cardiac output
- ❑ Improved cholesterol levels
- ❑ Improved immune function
- ❑ Improved sleep
- ❑ Improved vision
- ❑ Lowered blood pressure
- ❑ Mood elevation
- ❑ Reduction of cellulite
- ❑ Reduction of wrinkles
- ❑ Re-growth of hair
- ❑ Re-growth of shrunken organs
- ❑ Stronger bones
- ❑ Tighter, thicker, more hydrated skin
- ❑ PLUS: Enhancement of effects generated by replacement of other hormones

WHEN TO START HGH

The original studies on hGH were performed on men aged seventy to seventy-two. As a result, many physicians and their patients regard this general period as the appropriate time to start hGH replacement. But more recent data now indicates that the optimum time to start is much earlier. And it makes sense. Why start hGH therapy after all the damage has been done?

Early physical signs of growth-hormone deficiency include skeletal muscle loss, as evidenced by sagging skin in the face, arms, and buttocks. These signs are normally seen as people enter their fifties, and are often pronounced by the time they reach sixty. The blood test known as IGF-1 is an excellent indicator of your level of growth hormone. Optimum levels of IGF-1 should be greater than 200 ng/ml.

My IGF-1 levels dipped all the way down to 54 ng/ml when I was fifty-three. I was just starting to experience some of the signs and symptoms of growth-hormone deficiency at the time, so I was not all that surprised. I am 61 years old now and have been on growth-hormone replacement for eight years. The problems I was beginning to experience are simply gone. My current IGF-1 level is maintained at 300 ng/ml.

HOW ROBERT GOT BACK THE USE OF HIS KNEES

When Robert first came to me, he was sixty-two years old. Years of hard living had resulted in both good and bad effects. He had been a hard drinker until he was fifty-five, at which time he realized it was a problem and stopped. He told me, "I've never been happier in my whole life than I have been since I stopped drinking. The older I got, the more I realized how important my kids are to me, and the drinking was ruining my relationships."

On the good side of the equation was the fact that he had been a rancher all his life. He had always eaten real food, and had spent hours each day doing hard work. He appeared thin and reasonably healthy, but he looked about ten years older than his stated age—all the years of drinking had definitely accelerated the aging process for him.

He was complaining of moodiness, no sex drive, and insomnia. He also said he just did not have the energy to work around the ranch the way he used to. He was only sleeping five to six hours "on a good night," but his major concern was his knees. "An orthopedist told me my knees had been so deteriorated over the years, from arthritis and hard work, that the only solution available was joint replacement." Indeed, as he struggled to get out of the waiting room chair and then walk slowly into my office, it was apparent that his knees were a serious impediment.

Robert's symptoms were so characteristic of testosterone deficiency that I didn't even wait to get the tests back before starting him on replacement therapy. I also got him on QuickStart, DHEA, lipoic acid, and a low dose of thyroid. I also made sure he was following all the other important steps outlined in this book.

When he returned six weeks later to go over the test results, he was already starting to notice more energy, but his other symptoms were still very much in evidence. His tests revealed that he was extremely deficient in growth hormone. After I explained the many beneficial effects of hGH to him, he agreed to give it a try.

Two months later, he reported back that, "My energy level is starting to get much closer to the way it has always been, and best of all I am starting to really sleep well." He also said his knees were starting to feel better, and I noted how much more quickly he was able to get out of the chair.

Six months down the road, after nine months of therapy, he was "feeling as good as I ever had in my life, maybe even better." Particularly important was the fact that his knees were almost back to complete functioning. He was walking normally, and was able to hike up hills he hadn't even considered in years.

Robert's case is an excellent example of two important effects of hGH replacement. First, many of the beneficial effects of testosterone and DHEA replacement simply will not occur in the absence of adequate growth-hormone replacement. (Testosterone is a hormone that requires the presence of growth hormone in order to be fully effective.) Second, growth hormone can literally regenerate the lost cartilage in knees damaged by years of osteoarthritis and wear and tear.

The effects of hGH are mediated primarily through the action of the liver—once again, the all-important liver. For this reason, I recommend that anyone using hGH be sure to also include all the vitamins, minerals, and herbal supplements found in QuickStart. This, along with the other steps in this book, will guarantee optimal liver function.

In some cases, I also recommend hGH *stimulators*. These are specific amino acids that promote the secretion of hGH from the pituitary. Please note, however, that the response to these stimulators is modest and quite variable—as a rule, these agents usually have no significant effect in the over-fifty age group.

There is advertising of various brands of so-called homeopathic growth-hormone products sold on the Internet and in stores. These products, often sublingual sprays, purport to have growth hormone in them. Avoid them. They are worthless. Any benefit from them is purely placebo. All the medical studies showing benefits from hGH therapy have involved the injectable form of the hormone, and this is what I prescribe for my interested patients.

MELATONIN—MORE THAN JUST FOR SLEEPING

As a result of front-cover magazine treatment and the 1995 bestseller, *The Melatonin Miracle*, most people have heard about this celebrated hormone. And most of these people think of melatonin as a sleeping and jet-lag aid, which it certainly is. But its influence extends far beyond putting you to sleep. Let me cover a bit of the sleep connection first and then move on to the other exciting effects of melatonin.

Studies have shown a consistent and progressive decline in melatonin production starting in the early twenties. By age fifty, your melatonin level is half what it was in your early adult years. By seventy, it is less than half of what you had at fifty.

Is insomnia associated with aging? Yes, that's a direct effect of melatonin decline. Twenty-year-olds sleep an average of ten hours a night. Sixty-year-olds only get in six hours or so of sleep, much of it restless.

In 1995, one of the first scientific studies reporting this effect was published in the British medical journal, *The Lancet*. This was a double-blind placebo-controlled study, considered the most reliable kind of study design. The researchers demonstrated a direct relationship between the amount of melatonin being produced and the quality of sleep. They concluded that melatonin deficiency seems to be a key factor in the sleep disorders so common in older people.

Melatonin turns out to be a key element in the induction of a sleep cycle known as slow-wave sleep. This is the restorative stage of sleep when the body repairs the damage that has occurred during the day. Ever wonder why you don't heal as well from the stresses and strains of exercise or injury as you did when you were younger? You can blame much of that on a decreased level of melatonin. Austrian researchers have found that people who take a melatonin supplement spend a much longer time in slow-wave sleep than those who do not.

It is interesting to note that hGH is released by the pituitary during the slow-wave stage of sleep. A study published in the *Journal of the American Medical Association* (*JAMA*) revealed that sleep deprivation resulted in significantly lowered levels of growth-hormone production. This study once again serves to point out the close relationships between hormones.

The melatonin-sleeping connection, however, is really only the tip of the iceberg. There are many other talents of this extremely important hormone.

You've Got Rhythm

Melatonin is a major player, perhaps *the* major player, in your natural biological cycle known as the circadian rhythm, the inner intelligence that acts like a clock to control your sleep/wake cycle. Melatonin is secreted in the pineal gland, a part of the brain behind your forehead, which is extremely sensitive to sunlight. It releases melatonin in direct relationship to sunlight exposure. Sunlight causes the pineal gland to produce and store melatonon. When the sun sets and it becomes dark, the pineal gland releases the melatonin and induces the onset of sleep. This process regulates the circadian ryhthm.

I've covered the importance of obtaining adequate sunlight (*see* Chapter 10, Secret Three). Now here is another reason you need to get enough sun into your life.

The circadian rhythm is central to biological functioning. This fact was demonstrated by Walter Pierpaoli, M.D., the world-famous Italian researcher, in a series of dramatic and elaborate laboratory experiments in the early 1990s. Working with Vladimir Lesnikov, Ph.D., a Russian researcher, Pierpaoli surgically exchanged the pineal glands of young mice with those of old mice. Since the rodents were genetically identical, there was no rejection of the transplants.

As expected, the younger mice with the old pineal glands soon began to show the unmistakable signs of accelerated aging. Meanwhile, the older mice with the transplanted young glands appeared rejuvenated. At the end of the experiment, the old mice ended up living twice as long as the young ones. *In terms of human years, the old mice with the young glands lived more than one hundred years.* These experiments have led many experts in longevity medicine to regard melatonin as something of a fountain of youth.

Melatonin and Cancer

Some very convincing studies have shown that melatonin can help in the treatment and prevention of breast and prostate cancer. For example, in one study, researchers first grew estrogen-positive breast cancers in culture. They then supplied some of these cultures with the blood of women who had high levels of melatonin. The other cultures were exposed to the blood of women who had low levels of the hormone. What they found was striking.

When they were exposed to the lower levels of melatonin, the cancer cells divided much more rapidly. When the researchers spiked the low-melatonin blood samples with synthetic melatonin, it removed their capacity to promote cancer, and inhibited the growth of the cancer cells by 30–40 percent. According to one of the researchers, these results show "close to conclusively" that low melatonin levels promote breast-tumor growth.

It also shows that taking melatonin supplements may be effective in treating cancer. In one study published in the *British Journal of Cancer*, the use of melatonin supplements in women with breast cancer was effective in 28.5 percent of them. What is most impressive about this small study is that none of these women were responding to the conventional treatment they were getting.

Another study examined the levels of melatonin in the first morning urine of 147 women with invasive breast cancer and 291 women without cancer. They then combined both groups of women and noticed a distinct pattern dependent upon how high their melatonin levels were. Those in the highest melatonin group had close to one-half the risk of having breast cancer as those in the lowest group.

Since melatonin is formed during sleep, some other researchers took a slightly different approach. They looked at a group of 7,396 women over a period of six years. In this group, 146 women developed breast cancer. What they found was that those with the shortest amount of horizontal time, who, therefore, presumably had the lowest levels of melatonin, had almost three times the chance of developing cancer.

Other studies on melatonin and prostate cancer have been just as remarkable. Given these studies, it seems very prudent to supplement with melatonin once you hit your fifties.

Priming the Immune System

Melatonin also exerts a marked effect on the immune system. This is because melatonin enhances the immune activity of the thymus gland, located in the upper chest just below the neck. The thymus is a repository of first-line immune cells called lymphocytes. And it is here, in this gland, that immature lymphocytes go through a conditioning process—a kind of immune-system boot camp—that turns them into disease-fighting units that protect your body.

As people age, alas, the thymus gland atrophies and loses its ability to churn out mature immune cells called T-lymphocytes. This results in the lowered immune response so common in older people.

Receptor sites for melatonin have been found both on thymus cells and lymphocytes. In 1993, European researcher George Maestroni published the first study demonstrating that melatonin stimulated the production of T-lymphocytes in people with lowered immune function. He concluded that "the pineal gland might thus be viewed as the crux of a sophisticated immuno-neuroendocrine network."

But Wait—There's More

Melatonin also provides another major benefit to the body as an anti-oxidant. As previously discussed, free radicals create much, if not most, of the deterioration that occurs in the body as we age. Crucial antioxidant vitamins, such as vitamins C and E, along with CoQ_{10}, are the primary agents that snuff out harmful free-radical activity.

As an antioxidant, melatonin possesses its very own unique ability. An article by melatonin researcher R. Hardeland, which studied the antioxidant properties of melatonin, concluded that melatonin is an even more potent antioxidant than both vitamins C and E.

Additionally, researchers have also discovered that melatonin penetrates all the way into the nucleus of cells. There, it's antioxidant activity protects DNA from the type of free-radical destruction that can lead to cancer and neurological diseases. It is thought that melatonin may be able to limit the incidence of memory loss, Alzheimer's, and other brain disorders so common to older people.

According to Ray Sahelian, M.D., author of an excellent book, *Melatonin, Nature's Sleeping Pill*, "Melatonin, taken as a supplement, could slow down the aging process and decrease the incidences of brain damage and cancer."

I recommend starting melatonin supplementation around the age of fifty. This is when your body's production has started to go into a downslide. Try a small dose at first. I find that very little, half a milligram, is needed to maintain a youthful level. Even though very high doses of melatonin has been shown to be safe and non-toxic, they may cause sleep disturbances and morning drowsiness. Melatonin should be taken about half an hour before bedtime.

DHEA

Of all the hormones supplemented for anti-aging reasons, DHEA (dehydroepiandrosterone) is perhaps the best known. A lot has been written and said about it. Considerable research has been conducted showing that a low level of this adrenal hormone is associated with almost every disease studied. This list includes AIDS, Alzheimer's, cancer, cardiovascular disease, diabetes, lupus, osteoporosis, and viral and bacterial infections.

Clinically, I don't see the obvious and immediate benefit from DHEA replacement that I routinely observe with estrogen, hGH, progesterone, and testosterone therapy. Nevertheless, I regard DHEA as an extremely important element in a total disease-prevention strategy.

DHEA is the most abundant steroid hormone in the body. It is secreted in response to everything that stresses the body, from infections to allergies. By age seventy-five, however, you only produce about 10 percent of the amount you made as a twenty-five-year-old.

DHEA has been labeled as the *mother hormone*, because it can be, and often is, converted by the body into estrogen compounds and testosterone as they become low. The rate of this conversion differs widely among individuals and is significant enough that anyone taking DHEA needs to have these hormones monitored.

Many human studies involving DHEA supplementation mention the feeling of well-being that most people experience. I have found this generalized rejuvenating effect to be very consistent in my patients as well. I also see my older patients on DHEA recovering much more quickly from flu and colds. Only rarely do these infections last beyond a mild three or four days. This is partly attributable to DHEA's ability to boost the immune response in older people.

Animal studies have shown that DHEA protects the thymus gland from the normal shrinking that is associated with aging. This is the same thymus gland I mentioned in relation to melatonin, so here is another thymus-friendly hormone. Other promising animal studies have shown regression of tumors when animals were supplemented with DHEA.

My Recommendations to You

※ *If you are over forty,* look for a prevention-oriented physician familiar with natural hormonal testing and replacement therapy. He or she can gently and safely escort you into an effective program that will revitalize your life. *Do it now, even if you feel great.*

※ *The best treatment is prevention.* Don't wait until you are symptomatic. You can find a referral for an experienced practitioner near you by contacting the American Academy of Anti-Aging Medicine at www.world-health.net or by calling them at 773-528-1000.

☀ Use Bio-Energy Testing to determine your energy-production status. If your M-Factor (basal metabolism) is low, be sure your hormone replacement program includes thyroid. Rely on thyroid blood testing *only* to help monitor your replacement dosing. As I said, blood testing is useless for diagnosing low-thyroid states in most cases. That's why most Bio-Energy Testing is the best way to go. You can obtain a referral to a Bio-Energy Testing certified healthcare practitioner in your area by going to www.bioenergytesting.com or by calling 866-376-0610.

☀ Many natural hormones are available over the counter or through the Internet, but I always discourage people from getting their hormones this way. Many of the products are ineffective and some do not contain the potency they say they do. *A physician who is properly trained in natural bio-identical hormones is really necessary.* And through the doctor, and the compounding pharmacy she or he uses, you can purchase the very best quality of natural hormones.

☀ Because the hallmark of aging is a decreased E.Q., be sure that no matter how great you feel, your hormonal program optimizes your E.Q.

16

Putting It
All Together

I t's all about energy. How efficiently you produce it, and how efficiently your body uses what you produce. This book is all about how to maximize your energy production to youthful levels even as you get very old. In that way you will maintain your youthful strength and vigor, avoid disease, and age at the slowest possible rate. You will enjoy a much more functional, happy life. There are few things worse than growing old and being sick and dependent.

There's a huge amount of information in this book—and many guidelines. It's the same basic information I give my patients, only with them I don't have the time to go into all the detail I've included here. Don't be intimidated by everything you have read. Plan on incorporating this information into your life gradually over the next year. You will want to read the book several times, and earmark those sections that seem the most important to you. This is basic information. It will not grow old and obsolete with time. Certainly there will be many new and wonderful things to learn about in the years to come, but these basic tenets of health and longevity will always remain true.

I tell my patients I want them to eventually incorporate all the steps— all the secrets—into their everyday life. Bursting with energy isn't quite as simple as taking a single pill and voila—it's done. I wish it were, but it doesn't work that way. If I had that pill, I'd be the richest man in the world.

The anti-aging and detoxification program I've outlined is not just a temporary deal. It is an endeavor of a lifetime. And in order to live longer and healthier, the elements need to become routine. After saying this to my patients, I very quickly add that I don't want them to feel overwhelmed, so I encourage them to apply my guidelines sequentially—one at a time.

For the very best results, all the elements and steps I have discussed need to be addressed. That's because they work together. In other words, how you eat affects how you exercise, how you exercise affects how you sleep, how you sleep affects hormone production, and hormone production affects how you eat, exercise, and so forth.

In this book, I have laid out my recommendations—the secrets—in sequence, starting with the simplest steps. It's easy for instance, to start drinking more water, getting more rest, and going out into the sunlight. Those are my first three secrets.

Change is hard. Routine is easy. Once the changes I recommend become a part of your everyday life, they, too, will become routine and automatic. You will be replacing one routine for another one that is just as easy, but better for you. You can probably count on feeling some resistance at first, however, particularly if you are used to eating a certain way and are not used to exercising. But just focus on a three-month turnaround time. At the end of three months, the resistance will be gone, and will be replaced with the joy that accompanies feeling great.

Whatever it takes, just give yourself time to adopt the changes. Don't rush and try to accomplish all the steps too fast. It's not in your interest, or in the interest of the program, to become overwhelmed and stressed while trying to fashion a healthier lifestyle.

My supplement secret revolves mainly around my use of all the ingredients and doses in QuickStart and Super Fat. The breathing recommendations can be applied easily, and when practiced over time, can also become an automatic part of your life.

Hormone replacement can't be done on your own. You'll need to find a prevention and anti-aging specialist. To do that, contact either The American College for the Advancement of Medicine at 949-309-3520 (www.acam.org), or The American Academy of Anti-Aging Medicine at 773-528-1000 (www.worldhealth.net). These organizations can provide referrals.

Weight loss is always a tough nut to crack. But the information I have provided will give you a new perspective on why you may be having a harder time than necessary trying to lose weight. Hopefully, this information will provide new inspiration. If you are very overweight, this is something you cannot put off. It is too critical to your energy, longevity, and quality of life.

Ideally, you should start adopting all these guidelines as early as possible, and not wait until severe pain and debility make lifestyle changes that much more difficult to accomplish. But at any age, and in any condition, when these changes are made, they will bring fresh energy into your life. And if you are ailing, they will improve, perhaps even eliminate, your problem.

Make it a point to find a physician who can provide Bio-Energy Testing. It is the most amazing health-promoting technology I have ever encountered. It alone can pinpoint your energy-production deficits, and speed the process of overcoming them. If your doctor is not aware of Bio-Energy Testing, show him or her this book, and have them contact me through the phone numbers or website provided in Resources in back. You can also refer them to a very technical slide explanation of the entire testing process, which they can view at www.vrp.com/webinar/archive/. You might even want to see this slide presentation yourself. It is a one-hour lecture I gave in February of 2006 and the recording of it can be accessed free of charge at this site.

Let me say here, for the record, that I follow my own preaching. I know firsthand that it can be done. And that it is actually quite easy once you are used to it. I also know from my many patients that it works. When they follow the guidelines, their Bio-Energy Testing reveals energy levels that are typical of people much younger. They are literally bursting with energy.

Many of my recommendations are designed to make you feel better immediately, but a lot of what I say has prevention in mind. These preventive measures are also very, very important because, why would you want to feel better now, only to be sick later?

Medicine is changing as we speak. Soon, the days that seeing your doctor means you are sick will be gone. Now, physicians and their patients alike are finally getting the idea that seeing a doctor should be something you do *BEFORE* you are ill, in order to make sure you don't become ill.

If your physician is already familiar with this concept, great. This is important because you will not be able to implement some of the guidelines without the assistance of a prevention-oriented physician working with you.

GET AN ATTITUDE

Getting old is the perfect time to get a positive attitude. Enough cannot be said about the importance of attitude. I haven't talked about this so far because I wanted to save it for last, as it is probably the single most important component of life. *Your attitude can make or break anything else you do.* Attitude governs how happily or unhappily you live life—and perhaps how long you live it as well. I think you will agree that how long you live is really inconsequential compared to how well you live.

Did you hear the joke about the guy who goes in to see his doctor. After examining him, and checking out all the tests, the doctor says: "You're going to have to stop drinking, skiing, smoking cigars, and chasing women."

"Will it make me live longer, Doc?" the man asks.

"No, but I promise you it will make it seem longer."

Joking aside, I can promise you that sickness and pain will very definitely make life seem longer. And that, for sure, is not the quality of longevity you are seeking.

Growing old is just about the best thing that can happen to a person. It is a real gift. Make the most of it. Don't pay any attention to all the negative cultural messages implying you're over the hill. Sure, when you were younger maybe you could do things twice as fast, but you probably enjoyed them only half as much.

Don't yield to aging. The senior years represent the only time in your life when you are wise enough to really enjoy all that life has to offer. The key is, *while you grow old chronologically, you don't have to keep pace biologically.* You can have youthful energy levels, and feel great even at very old ages. That's what the book is about.

Nor do you have to grow old psychologically. Think young. Ask yourself, "Is there anything I would do now if I were only younger?" If there is a positive answer to this question, my advice to you is to do it. This is your life, live it to the fullest until it ends. Now is a great time to rid yourself of any negative attitudes and assumptions that get in the way.

Appreciate all your good qualities, and work on developing more. Accept full responsibility for every aspect of your life. For what has gone wrong. And for what has gone right. This is what free will is all about. The realization of this is the source of all your power, including the power to get well and stay well.

The four most important aspects of life are relationships, money, work, and health. All require some work. They are never dialed in. They constantly change, and must be continuously reexamined. Get some professional counseling if you need it. There is no one who can't benefit from counseling every now and then.

Happiness is not a goal. It's a pursuit. And so is contentment in who you are, and how you live your life. Don't compare yourself to others, it's a waste of valuable time. There will always be someone who is better, and someone who is worse, so what's the point?

Whenever you can, sing, dance, pray, rejoice, and laugh—especially at yourself. Don't you sometimes feel like one of the Three Stooges, only without the sophistication? Be forgiving with yourself. If you don't forgive yourself, you won't be able to forgive others.

Lastly, don't be afraid to try on new attitudes. It's OK to make mistakes at any age. Mistakes are how we learn. They actually aren't mistakes, they are lessons. You get them over and over until you learn. If you don't learn, you don't grow. Imagine how smart you're going to be after an entire lifetime of lessons.

Good Luck!

Dr. Shallenberger's Super Immune QuickStart Plus Super Fat Ingredients

Dr. Shallenberger is licensed both as a Medical Doctor and a Homeopathic Medical Doctor, and has been practicing nutritional and preventive medicine since 1978. During that time, he has analyzed the biochemical and nutritional needs of literally thousands of his patients. He discovered there were certain nutrients and herbs that all his patients needed, and he decided to put full doses of all these ingredients in one easy-to-take product.

While it is in no way a substitution for a healthy diet, the spectrum and doses in this mixture reflect the current state of the art in nutritional supplementation and detoxification. When used in conjunction with Super Fat and a three-week detoxification program of exercise and abstention from alcohol, coffee, flour, milk, and sweets, Dr. Shallenberger's QuickStart formula prevents and often solves many problems and disorders without any other intervention needed.

PILLS VS. FOOD

Because of the complex nature of digestive tracts, capsules and tablets are not the best way of delivering nutrients. There are four basic reasons for this.

First, some vitamin content may be decreased in the manufacturing process.

Second, tablets and capsules do not always adequately break down in many people, which means that much of their content may not be absorbed.

Third, it would require over sixty horse-size capsules to get the same amount of nutrients found in the recommended amount of QuickStart. Very few people are going to take that many capsules for very long, if they would even take them in the first place.

Four, Dr. Shallenberger has carefully formulated this product so that each vitamin, mineral, and herb is present in the exact form he has determined to be the most clinically effective.

All the nutrients in QuickStart are prepared as a fine powder. Not only are nutrient values maintained throughout the manufacturing process, but also the absorption rate is high, even in individuals with compromised digestive systems.

IMMUNE SYSTEMS UNDER SIEGE

What causes one person to catch a flu and another to avoid it? Why does one person develop an immune-related disease while another living in the same environment doesn't? Why do some people have allergies? Why do serious outbreaks of infectious diseases leave some individuals untouched? The answers, of course, live within the immune system.

From viruses never before discovered to antibiotic-resistant bacteria, immune systems are being challenged in ways never before seen. These times require the most supercharged immune systems imaginable. Through diet, adequate rest, and the special nutrients in Dr. Shallenberger's formula, you will harness your body's ability to do the job that nature intended —combat and prevent disease.

THE ULTIMATE PRESCRIPTION

Many people taking QuickStart have reported a noticeable improvement in a variety of conditions, despite the fact that QuickStart was often the only clinical intervention they were using. This is because the formula works on such basic levels, providing antioxidant protection and nutritional insurance, while at the same time enhancing immunity, alkalinizing tissues, improving brain function, improving circulation, detoxifying the liver and intestinal tract, stabilizing appetite and metabolism, and, most importantly, increasing energy production.

Consultants will appreciate the fact that QuickStart is not just another multi-vitamin using meaningless doses of many nutrients merely to make the label look good. Every ingredient is clinically proven, and is added in its full recommended amount.

QuickStart is the only product available that has the recommended amount of *all* the vitamins, minerals, and antioxidants, in addition to the full-strength detoxifying power of rice bran, psyllium, n-acetyl cysteine, l-glutamine, and spirolina Pacifica. QuickStart also contains the hormone-balancing effects of soy protein isolates, the remarkable immune-enhancing power of astragalus and hydrolized whey protein, and the prostate and breast-cancer prevention afforded by saw palmetto extract. Additionally, QuickStart offers the blood thinning and circulation enhancement power of ginkgo biloba extract.

QUICKSTART INGREDIENTS

Two Scoops (42.3 grams) provides:

* 30,000 IU beta carotene
* 10,000 IU vitamin A
* 2,000 mg vitamin C
* 400 IU vitamin E (d-alpha)
* 1000 mg Hesperidin Bioflav Complex
* 120 mg ginkgo biloba extract
* 600 mg magnesium (citrate)
* 10 mg manganese (amino-acid chelate)
* 300 mg potassium (citrate)
* 200 mcg selenium (selenate)
* 1200 mcg chromium (picolinate)
* 16 mg zinc (picolinate)
* 2 mg copper (amino-acid chelate)
* 100 mg vitamin B_1

* 50 mg vitamin B_2
* 100 mg niacin
* 300 mg pantothenic acid
* 100 mg vitamin B_6
* 1000 mcg vitamin B_{12}
* 1000 mcg folic acid
* 500 mcg biotin
* 300 mg astragalus extract
* 6 gm spirolina Pacifica
* 750 mg L-glutamine
* 100 mg n-acetyl cysteine (NAC)
* 320 mg saw palmetto
* 5 gm psyllium husks
* 5 gm stabilized rice bran
* 5 gm soy protein isolate*
* 5 gm whey protein (undenatured)*

* Note: Some people are allergic to soy or whey. For them, there is QuickStart-HA (hypo-allergenic). QuickStart-HA provides the same nutrients found in regular QuickStart, but hypo-allergenic rice protein is substituted for the soy and whey protein content.

SUPER FAT INGREDIENTS

One teaspoon provides:

- ☀ 3 cc fish oil concentrate
- ☀ 1 cc wheat germ oil
- ☀ 1 cc flax oil
- ☀ 135 mg mixed tocopherols, containing 20 percent gamma tocopherol

- ☀ 15 mg lycopene
- ☀ 50 mg CoQ_{10}
- ☀ 50 mg lipoic acid
- ☀ 750 mg vitamin D_3

DIRECTIONS

At first, start taking QuickStart as a breakfast replacement in the morning, and again as an adrenal supporter in the afternoon, sometime between noon and 3 PM. It usually takes a few weeks to get into the habit of remembering this afternoon dose, but once you see how much your energy levels improve, it will become second nature.

Always start with a half scoop or less. The formula is quite strong, and it may take up to a week for the liver to adjust to QuickStart. After you have adjusted to the starting amount, gradually increase to the recommended amount of one scoop.

Although QuickStart can be taken simply by shaking it up with water, many people enjoy making a smoothie by adding extras such as vanilla, yogurt, or fruit, along with water and ice, and blending it in a blender. Be sure to also add half a teaspoon of Super Fat to the morning dose.

HOW TO ORDER QUICKSTART

QuickStart can be ordered by calling the toll-free number 866-376-0610. It can also be ordered online at www.bioenergytesting.com.

As per federal guidelines, we need to inform you that these statements have not been evaluated by the FDA. This product is not intended to diagnose, treat, or cure any disease. If you are sick please consult a physician.

APPENDIX B

Is Your Patient Exercising Too Hard To Be Healthy?

FRANK SHALLENBERGER, MD, HMD, ABAAM

TOWNSEND LETTER FOR DOCTORS.
August/September, 2004, 97–99.

Abstract

Context: Aerobic exercise is a documented and well-accepted measure to decrease incidence of degenerative disease, increase quality of life, and extend lifespan. However, exercising above anaerobic threshold is known to increase free-radical production, and exhaust both redox buffering and acid-base buffering capabilities. Both of these phenomena are known to increase the rate of aging and tissue and organ degeneration. It is not clear whether exercising at levels of exertion consistent with the most popular current method of predicting anaerobic threshold is healthy.

Objective: To examine if the predictive formula, anaerobic-threshold heart rate = .8 × (220 − age), is a safe formula to use in prescribing an exercise regimen for health and longevity.

Design, Setting, and Participants: Nineteen patients who were free of degenerative disease, and who were consulting a board-certified physician in anti-aging medicine for purposes of longevity and disease prevention were randomly selected. Patients served as their own controls.

Main Outcome Measure: Heart rate at anaerobic threshold as determined, using respiratory gas-exchange analysis and a computer-driven algorithm known as Bio-Energy Testing.

Results: Among nineteen patients tested, sixteen (84%) had a measured anaerobic-threshold heart rate which was significantly below, and two (10%) had a measured anaerobic-threshold heart rate which was significantly above that predicted by the formula, anaerobic-threshold heart rate = .8 x (220-age). Thirteen (68%) had a measured anaerobic-threshold heart which was at least 10% less than that predicted by the formula. Furthermore, the point of anaerobic threshold could not be accurately determined by the classical clinical symptoms of anaerobic threshold, such as significant breathlessness and muscle pain.

Conclusion: Using either the predictive formula: anaerobic-threshold heart rate = .8 $\times$ (220 − age), or the clinical signs of breathlessness and muscle pain to prescribe an exercise regimen for health and longevity is unreliable, and in the majority of cases will result in patients exercising at dangerously high levels.

INTRODUCTION

Aerobic exercise is a documented and well-accepted measure to decrease incidence of degenerative disease, increase quality of life, and extend lifespan.[1,2] As the intensity of exercise increases, the rate of oxygen consumption increases in order to provide the necessary energy production for the increased exertional demand. In any given subject, as the intensity of exertion is steadily and incrementally increased, he will eventually come to a level of exertion which exceeds his body's capacity to consume oxygen. This point is referred to as the subject's anaerobic threshold because, if the level of exertion is increased beyond this point, he will no longer be able to meet his energy needs from oxygen metabolism, and he will begin to produce energy anaerobically.

It is important for every person who exercises to know at what level of exertion he will exceed his oxygen-consuming capacity and enter into anaerobic metabolism because anaerobic metabolism is known to dramatically increase the production of powerful pro-oxidant molecules known as free radicals. Many, if not most, of the damaging effects that occur during the aging process and in degenerative disease are mediated by free radicals.[3] Most of these free radicals are eliminated by antioxidant enzyme buffering systems, such as glutathione peroxidase, catalase, and superoxide dismutase, but in the process of eliminating free-radical stress, these enzymes are consumed. Sustained exertional effort above anaerobic threshold produces such an abundance of free radicals that these redox buffering enzymes eventually become depleted.[4] This depletion results in an increased rate of aging and risk of disease secondary to increased oxidant stress.

Furthermore, exercising above the anaerobic threshold also produces an abundance of lactic acid. The lactic acid is either recycled in the Cori cycle, in which it is converted in the liver back into glucose, converted into carbon dioxide through the action of the enzyme carbonic anhydrase, or buffered by various acid-base buffering systems. The first two of these systems has limitations however.

The Cori system requires ATP, which results in increased energy consumption at a time when energy needs are already being exceeded. The carbonic anhydrase system is limited by respiration, which is evidenced by the fact that as a subject exceeds his anaerobic threshold, his serum levels of both carbon dioxide and lactate increase. Because of these limitations, sustained exercise above anaerobic threshold results in increased demands on the acid-base buffering systems, which eventually depletes these systems. Similar to what happens when antioxidant buffering is depleted, a depletion of acid-base buffering results in a sustained increase in mesenchymal acid levels. Increased mesenchymal acidosis is known to dramatically mediate both acute and chronic disease as well as most of the pathology associated with the aging process.[5]

Thus, exercising above anaerobic threshold results in an increase in oxidant stress as well as an increase in mesenchymal acidosis, and both of these phenomena increase the rate of aging and tissue and organ degeneration. Ironically enough, many people who exercise regularly may be actually increasing their rate of aging if they are exercising above their anaerobic threshold. This fact is well known, and to avoid doing so, subjects are advised to use the following formula to determine what their heart rate will be as they come close to their anaerobic threshold:

$$\text{Anaerobic-threshold heart rate} = .8 \times (220 - \text{age})$$

Subjects are commonly advised to use this formula to avoid exercising above this determined heart rate in order to avoid exceeding their anaerobic threshold. Furthermore, many exercise experts feel that a subject will immediately sense when he is exceeding his anaerobic threshold because the increased production of lactic acid will result in noticeable muscle pain along with a very noticeable increase in respiration. The objective of this experiment was to determine the following:

1. Is the formula, anaerobic-threshold heart rate = .8 × (220 − age), accurate in predicting the point at which a subject enters into anaerobic metabolism?

2. Is the presence of muscle pain and/or significant breathlessness accurate in predicting the point at which a subject enters into anaerobic metabolism?

If these predictors, which are so commonly used, are not accurate, then many people may be exercising *too hard to be healthy.*

METHODS

Nineteen healthy patients who were free of disease, and who were consulting a board-certified physician in anti-aging medicine for purposes of longevity and disease prevention were randomly selected. Ages varied from nineteen to seventy-one. Patients served as their own controls.

Oxygen consumption and carbon-dioxide production were determined using a pulmonary gas analyzer and an exercise ergometer supplied by Medical Graphics Corporation, St. Paul, MN. This equipment uses a mouthpiece which analyzes all of a subject's inspired and expired air for oxygen and carbon-dioxide content. Oxygen consumption and carbon-dioxide production were determined on each patient while exercising on the ergometer. The workload of the ergometer was steadily increased at varying rates, using a protocol provided by Bio-Energy Testing, LLC, Carson City, NV, which is based on a predicted level of fitness for each patient. The test was concluded as soon as the patient reached his anaerobic threshold.

The breath-by-breath data, consisting of oxygen consumption, carbon-dioxide production, and heart rate, were analyzed by a patented computer-driven algorithm, Bio-Energy Testing, provided by Bio-Energy Testing, LLC. Anaerobic threshold was determined by this algorithm to occur when the rate of oxygen consumption is exceeded by the rate of carbon-dioxide production. The point at which the rate of oxygen consumption is exceeded by the rate of carbon-dioxide production is generally accepted as the most accurate determination of anaerobic threshold.[6] The heart rate, when the anaerobic threshold was reached, was then reported as True Anaerobic-Threshold Heart Rate (TATR).

The patient's age was then used to estimate the heart rate at which anaerobic threshold would be reached according to the formula, anaerobic-threshold heart rate $= .8 \times (220 - \text{age})$. This heart rate was reported as Estimated Anaerobic-Threshold Heart Rate (EATR).

RESULTS

Full results are shown in Table 1. Among nineteen patients tested, sixteen (84%) had a TATR which was significantly below EATR. Thirteen (68%) had a TATR which was at least 10% below EATR, a point which is considered as an extremely conservative estimation of anaerobic-threshold heart rate. Two (10%) had a TATR which was significantly above the patient's EATR.

Only in two cases did the point of anaerobic threshold coincide with the classical clinical symptoms of anaerobic threshold, such as significant breathlessness and muscle pain. This occurred only in the two patients in which the TATR was significantly above the patient's EATR.

CONCLUSION

Using either the predictive formula, anaerobic-threshold heart rate $= .8 \times (220 - \text{age})$, or the clinical signs of breathlessness and muscle pain to estimate anaerobic-threshold heart rate was unreliable in 100% of patients tested. Exercise programs prescribed on the basis of this formula and these symptoms will result in 90% of patients exercising above their aerobic capacity, which will thus expose these patients to dangerously high levels of oxidant stress and mesenchymal acidosis. Even more ominous is the fact that, when using these criteria, 68% of patients will be exercising 10–25 percent above their anaerobic threshold.

DISCUSSION

That anaerobic threshold can be determined by pulmonary gas analysis is well established.[6] It occurs at the point in which lactic-acid production becomes greatly accelerated due to the fact that, since energy needs can no longer be met by aerobic mechanisms, they must be met by anaerobic metabolism. In order to produce the same amount of ATP as aerobic metabolism, anaerobic metabolism must produce more than eighteen times the amount of lactic acid. Through the action of the enzyme carbonic anhydrase, the increasing levels of lactic acid are converted to carbon dioxide in order to avoid sustained metabolic acidosis. This increase in carbon dioxide can be measured in the expired pulmonary gases. Anaerobic threshold occurs when the levels of carbon dioxide exceed the rate of oxygen consumption.[6]

Although many studies have shown that increased total time exercising results in better health outcomes, there is evidence that overly intense exercise programs may be harmful.[7,8,9,10] This study demonstrates why. It is because the majority of people who exercise in America are not in a high enough level of fitness to perform intense exercise. For them, intense exercise, as is predicted by breathlessness and the predictive formula commonly used by exercise trainers, only results in increased oxidant stress and mesenchymal acidosis. Ironically enough, this is exactly what they are exercising to avoid. No doubt this is why the majority of people who enter into an exercise regime, either on their own or under the guidance of a fitness trainer, eventually stop the program. On some level, they realize it is not good for them.

Only two people in this study had an anaerobic threshold that was not below the predicted value. Both of these people were competitive athletes, and for them the predicted anaerobic threshold was too low. Using that model, they would not have been exercising to their maximum aerobic capacity, and thus not exercising efficiently.

Therefore, in this study of nineteen healthy subjects, the predictive formula studied was in significant error 100% of the time. We conclude that this formula is essentially useless. Furthermore, even when the more conservative formula, anaerobic-threshold heart rate $= .6 \times (220 - \text{age})$, is used, over 68% of the patients will still be exercising above their predicted aerobic capacity.

Based on this study, physicians should only be prescribing exercise programs based upon the true anaerobic threshold, as determined by individual measurement. This can be easily and accurately determined using a combination of a pulmonary gas analyzer and a computer program (Bio-Energy Testing) designed to determine the level at which carbon-dioxide production exceeds oxygen consumption.

NAME	AGE	ESTIMATED ATR	TRUE ATR	TATR/EATR
Lawrance	67	130	97	–26%
Chuck	47	147	122	–18%
Miguel	19	170	136	–20%
Larry	58	137	136	n.s.
Joseph	68	129	105	–19%
Larry	60	136	115	–16%
John	71	126	109	–14%
Heinz	59	136	123	–10%
Karen	54	141	148	+4%
Alice	42	151	148	–2%
Karen	39	153	126	–18%
Maureen	50	144	135	–7%
Joy	69	128	112	–13%
Lauren	20	170	150	–12%
Alice	58	137	116	–16%
Cathie	52	142	119	–17%
Margaret	71	126	120	–5%
Susan	65	131	114	–13%
Frank	56	139	160	+15%

Highlighted TATR/EATR values represent patients who would have been exercising at least 10% over their anaerobic threshold if the estimated heart-rate formula had been applied. This is a point which is considered an extremely conservative estimation of anaerobic-threshold heart rate.

References

1. Lee, IM, Hsieh, CC, Paffenbarger, RS. "Exercise intensity and longevity in men." The Harvard Alumni Health Study. *Journal of the American Medical Association (JAMA)*. 273(15):1179–1184, Apr 19, 1995.

2. Jones TF, Eaton, CB. "Exercise prescription." *American Family Physician*. 52(2):543–550, 553–555, Aug 1995.

3. Harman, D. "Free radicals and the origin, evolution, and present status of the free radical theory of aging." *Free Radicals in Molecular Biology, Aging, and Disease*, ed. D. Armstrong et al. New York, NY: Raven, 1984.

4. Levine, SA, Kidd, PM. "Antioxidant Adaptation—its role in free-radical pathology." Biocurrents Division, San Leandro, CA., 1982.

5. Pischinger, A. *Matrix and Matrix Regulation*. Haug International, Brussels, 1975.

6. Wasserman, K, Hansen, JE, et al. *Principles of Exercise Testing and Interpretation*. Lippincott, Williams, and Wilkins, 1999.

7. Sherman, SE, D'Agostino, RB, Cobb, JL, Kannel, WB. "Does exercise reduce mortality rates in the elderly?" Experience from the Framingham Heart Study. *American Heart Journal*. 128(5):965–977, Nov 1994.

8. Lee, IM, Skerrett, PJ. "Physical activity and all-cause mortality: what is the dose-response relation?" *Medicine and Science in Sports and Exercise*. 33(6 Suppl):S459–471; discussion S493–494, Jun 2001.

9. Shephard, RJ. "Absolute versus relative intensity of physical activity in a dose-response context. *Medicine and Science in Sports and Exercise*. 33(6 Suppl):S400–418; discussion S419–420, Jun 2001.

10. Smekal, G, Pokan, R, Baron, R, et al. "Amount and intensity of physical exercise in primary prevention." *Wiener Medizinische Wochenschrift*. 151(1–2):7–12, 2001.

Resources

American Academy of Anti-Aging Medicine
1510 W. Montana Street
Chicago, IL 60614
Ph: 773-528-1000
Fax: 773-528-5390
Website: www.worldhealth.net
e-mail: info@worldhealth.net

American College for the Advancement of Medicine
24411 Ridge Route, Suite 115
Laguna Hills, CA 92653
Ph: 949-309-3520 or 800-532-3688
Fax: 949-309-3538
Website: www.acam.org
e-mail: info@acam.org

Bio-Energy Testing System
1231 Country Club Drive
Carson City, Nevada 89703
Ph: 866-376-0610
Fax: 775-884-2202
Website: www.bioenergytesting.com
e-mail: nvcenter@nvbell.net

Bio-Energy Testing centers are now being established throughout the United States and the world. A current list of centers using Bio-Energy Testing can be found at the website listed above. We invite doctors, healthcare practitioners, and fitness centers to inquire about offering this test for their clients.

**Dr. Shallenberger and The Nevada Center
of Alternative and Anti-Aging Medicine**
1231 Country Club Drive
Carson City, Nevada, 89703
Ph: 775-884-3990
Fax: 775-884-2202
Website: www.antiagingmedicine.com
e-mail: nvcenter@nvbell.net
       Doctors: doctor@bioenergytesting.com
       Sales: nvcntrji@nvbell.net

References

Chapter 2

Bliznakov, EG, Watanabe, T, Saji, S, et al. "Coenzyme Q deficiency in aged mice." *Journal of Medicine.* 9(4):337–346, 1978.

Blomstrand, R, Diczfalusy, U, Sisfontes, L, et al. "Influence of dietary partially hydrogenated vegetable and marine oils on membrane composition and function of liver microsomes and platelets in the rat." Lipids. 20(5):283–295, May 1985.

De Schrijver, R, Privett, OS. "Energetic efficiency and mitochondrial function in rats fed trans fatty acids." *Journal of Nutrition.* 114(7):1183–1191, Jul 1984.

Etzioni, A, Levy, J, Nitzan, M, et al. "Systemic carnitine deficiency exacerbated by a strict vegetarian diet." *Archives of Disease in Childhood.* 59(2):177–179, Feb 1984.

Kummerow, FA. "Dietary effects of trans fatty acids." *Journal of Environmental Pathology, Toxicology, and Oncology.* 6(3-4):123–149, Mar–Apr 1986.

Lombard, KA, Olson, AL, Erde, P, et al. "Carnitine status of lactoovovegetarians and strict vegetarian adults and children." *American Journal of Clinical Nutrition.* 50(2):301–306, Aug 1989.

Mozaffarian, D, Katan, MB, Ascherio, A et al. "Trans Fatty Acids and Cardiovascular Disease." *New England Journal of Medicine.* 354(15):1601–1613, PMID 16611951, April 2006.

National Academies Press. "Dietary Reference Intakes for Energy, Carbohydrate, Fiber, Fat, Fatty Acids, Cholesterol, Protein, and Amino Acids (Macronutrients)." 2005, 1.

Ravaglia, G, Forti, P, Maioli, F, et al. "Effect of micronutrient status on natural killer cell immune function in healthy free-living subjects." *American Journal of Clinical Nutrition.* 71(2):590–598, Feb 2000.

Chapter 3

Beal, MF. "Mitochondria, oxidative damage, and inflammation in Parkinson's disease." *Annals of the New York Academy of Science.* 991:120–131. Review, Jun 2003.

Caldwell, SH, Chang, CY, Nakamoto, RK, et al. "Mitochondria in nonalcoholic fatty liver disease." *Clinical Liver Disease.* 8(3):595–617, Aug 2004.

Duchen, MR. "Mitochondria in health and disease: perspectives on a new mitochondrial biology." *Molecular Aspects of Medicine.* 25(4):365–451, Aug 2004.

Hagen, TM, Ingersoll, RT, et al. "Acetyl-L-carnitine fed to old rats partially restores mitochondrial function and ambulatory activity." Proceedings of the National Academy of Sciences. USA. 95 (16):9562–9566, Aug 4, 1998.

Hagen, TM, Liu, J, et al. "Feeding acetyl-L-carnitine and lipoic acid to old rats significantly improves metabolic function while decreasing oxidative stress." Proceedings of the National Academy of Sciences. USA. 99:1870–1875, Feb 19, 2002.

Klatz, R, Goldman, R. *Stopping the Clock.* New Canaan, CT: Keats Publishing, Inc. 1997.

Krieger, C, Duchen, MR. "Mitochondria, Ca2+ and neurodegenerative disease." *European Journal of Pharmacology.* 447(2–3):177–188. Review, Jul 5, 2002.

Lamson, DW, Plaza, SM. "Mitochondrial factors in the pathogenesis of diabetes: a hypothesis for treatment." *Alternative Medical Review.* 7(2):94–111. Review, Apr 2002.

Lee, HC, Wei, YH. "Mitochondrial alterations, cellular response to oxidative stress and defective degradation of proteins in aging." *Biogerontology.* 2(4):231–244, 2001.

Lesnefsky, EJ, Hoppel, CL. "Ischemia-reperfusion injury in the aged heart: role of mitochondria." *Archives of Biochemical Biophysics.* 15;420(2):287–297. Review, Dec 2003.

Shallenberger, Frank. *Practicing Anti-Aging Medicine In The New Millenium.* First International Learning Conference on Anti-Aging Medicine in Monte Carlo, Monaco. June 24, 2000.

Speakman, JR, Talbot, DA, et al. "Uncoupled and surviving: individual mice with high metabolism have greater mitochondrial uncoupling and live longer." *Aging Cell.* 3(3):87–95, Jun 2004.

Trifunovic, A, Wredenberg, A, et al. "Premature aging in mice expressing defective mitochondrial DNA polymerase." *Nature.* 429(6990):417–423, May 27, 2004.

Trounce, I, Byrne, E, Marzuki, S. "Decline in skeletal muscle mitochondrial respiratory chain function: possible factor in aging." *The Lancet.* 25;1(8639):637–639, Mar 1989.

Wenzel, U, Nickel, A, Daniel, H. "Increased carnitine-dependent fatty acid uptake into mitochondria of human colon cancer cells induces apoptosis." *Journal of Nutrition.* 35(6):1510–1514, Jun 1, 2005.

Wilson, TM, Tanaka, H. "Meta-analysis of the age-associated decline in maximal aerobic capacity in men: relation to training status." *The American Journal of Physiology.* 278: 829–834, 2000.

Chapter 4

Abraham, AS, Sonnenblick, M, Eini, M. "The effect of chromium on cholesterol-induced atherosclerosis in rabbits." *Atherosclerosis.* 41(2–3):371–379, Feb 1982.

Banerjee, S, Crook, AM, Dawson, JR, et al. "Magnitude and consequences of error in coronary angiography interpretation (the ACRE study)." *American Journal of Cardiology.* 85(3):309–314, Feb 1, 2000.

Cantin, B, et al. "Lipoprotein (a) Distribution in a French Canadian Population and Its Relation to Intermittent Claudication." (The Quebec Cardiovascular Study)." *American Journal of Cardiology.* 75:1224–1228, 1995.

Cantorna, MT, Zhu, Y, Froicu, M, et al. "Vitamin D status, 1,25-dihydroxyvitamin D_3, and the immune system." *American Journal of Clinical Nutrition.* 80(6 Suppl):1717S–1720S, Dec; 2004.

Fenech, M. "Chromosomal damage rate, aging, and diet." *Annals of the New York Academy of Sciences.* 854:23–36, Nov 20, 1998.

Frick, MH, Elo, O, Haapa, K, et al. "Helsinki Heart Study: primary-prevention trial with gemfibrozil in middle-aged men with dyslipidemia. Safety of treatment, changes in risk factors, and incidence of coronary heart disease." *New England Journal of Medicine.* 317(20):1237–1245, Nov 2, 1987.

Gavish, D, et al. "Lipoprotein (a) reduction by N-Acetyl-cysteine." *The Lancet.* 337:203–204, 1991.

Gaziano, JM, Hennekens, CH, O'Donnell, CJ, et al. "Fasting triglycerides, high-density lipoprotein, and risk of myocardial infarction." *Circulation.* 96(8):2520–2525, Oct 21, 1997.

Giovannucci, E, Rimm, EB, Wolk, A, et al. "Calcium and fructose intake in relation to risk of prostate cancer." *Cancer Research.* 58(3):442–447, Feb 1, 1998.

Guadagnoli, E, Hauptman, PJ, Ayanian, JZ, et al. "Variation in the use of cardiac procedures after acute myocardial infarction." *New England Journal of Medicine.* 333(9):573–578, Aug 31, 1995.

Horner, SM. "Efficacy of intravenous magnesium in acute myocardial infarction in reducing arrhythmias and mortality. Meta-analysis of magnesium in acute myocardial infarction." *Circulation.* 86(3):774–779, Sept, 1992.

Isidoro, A, Martinez, M, Fernandez, PL, et al. "Alteration of the bioenergetic phenotype of mitochondria is a hallmark of breast, gastric, lung and oesophageal cancer." *Biochemistry Journal.* 378(Pt 1):17–20, Feb 15, 2004.

Jackson, RD, LaCroix, AZ, Gass, M, et al. "Calcium plus vitamin D supplementation and the risk of fractures." *New England Journal of Medicine.* 354(7): 669–683, Feb 16, 2006.

Mark, DB, Naylor, CD, Hlatky, MA, et al. "Use of Medical Resources and Quality of Life after Acute Myocardial Infarction in Canada and the United States." *New England Journal of Medicine.* 17(331):1130–1135. Oct 27, 1984.

Mayer-Davis, EJ, D'Agostino, R Jr, Karter, AJ, et al. "Intensity and amount of physical activity in relation to insulin sensitivity: the Insulin Resistance Atherosclerosis Study." *Journal of the American Medical Association (JAMA).* 279(9): 669–674, Mar 4, 1998.

Paterson, CR. "Calcium requirements in man: a critical review." *Postgraduate Medical Journal.* 54(630):244–248, Apr 1978.

Rifkind, BM. "Lipid Research Clinics Coronary Primary Prevention Trial: results and implications." *American Journal of Cardiology.* 54(5):30C–34C, Aug 27, 1984.

Schaefer, EJ, et al. "Lipoprotein (a) levels and risk of coronary heart disease in men." *Journal of the American Medical Association (JAMA).* 271(3):999–1003, 1994.

Schulz, TJ, Thierbach, R, et al. "Induction of oxidative metabolism by mitochondrial frataxin inhibits cancer growth: Otto Warburg revisited." *Journal of Biological Chemistry.* 281(2):977–981. Epub Nov 1, 2005, Jan 13, 2006.

Simonoff, M. "Chromium deficiency and cardiovascular risk. *Cardiovascular Research.* 18(10):591–596, Oct 1984.

Wallace, DC. "Mitochondria and cancer: Warburg addressed." Cold Spring Harbor Symposium on Quantitative Biology.70:363–374, 2005.

"WHO cooperative trial on primary prevention of ischaemic heart disease with clofibrate to lower serum cholesterol: final mortality follow-up." Report of the Committee of Principal Investigators. *The Lancet.* 2(8403):600–604, Sep 15, 1984.

"WHO cooperative trial on primary prevention of ischaemic heart disease using clofibrate to lower serum cholesterol: mortality follow-up." Report of the Committee of Principal Investigators. *The Lancet.* 2(8191):379–385, Aug 23, 1980.

Zucker, M. *User's Guide to Coenzyme Q_{10}.* North Bergen, NJ: Basic Health Publications, 2002.

Chapter 5

Liu, J, Atamna, H, Kuratsune, H, et al. "Delaying brain mitochondrial decay and aging with mitochondrial antioxidants and metabolites." *Annals of the New York Academy of Sciences.* 959:133–166, Apr 2002.

Chapter 6

Eggleston, DW. "Effect of dental amalgam and nickel alloys on T-lymphocytes: preliminary report." *Journal of Prosthetic Dentistry.* 51(5):617–623, May 1984.

Vimy, MJ, Lorscheider, FL. "Serial measurements of intra-oral air mercury: estimation of daily dose from dental amalgam." *Dental Research* 64:1072–1075, 1985.

Chapter 7

Daly, J. "The ventilatory response of exercise in CFS." The Third Annual Conference on Chronic Fatigue Syndrome and the Brain, Bel-Air, California, April 24–26, 1992.

Hagen, TM, Liu, J, Lykkesfeldt, J, et al. "Feeding acetyl-L-carnitine and lipoic acid to old rats significantly improves metabolic function while decreasing oxidative stress." *Proceedings of the National Academy of Science, USA.* 99(4): 1870–1875, Feb 19, 2002.

Shigenaga, MK, Hagen, TM, Ames, BN. "Oxidative damage and mitochondrial decay in aging." *Proceedings of the National Academy of Science, USA.* 91:10771–10778, Nov 1994.

Speakman, JR, Talbot, DA, et al. "Uncoupled and surviving: individual mice with high metabolism have greater mitochondrial uncoupling and live longer." *Aging Cell.* 3(3):87–95, Jun 2004.

Stevens, SR. "Using exercise testing to document functional disability in CFS." *Journal of Chronic Fatigue Syndrome.* 1(3/4):127–129, 1995.

Wasserman, K, Hansen, J, Sue, D, et al. *Principles of exercise testing and interpretation.* Third Edition, Lippincott, Williams, and Wilkins, Baltimore, MD, 1999, p. 18.

Chapter 8

Batmanghelidj, F. *Your Body's Many Cries for Water.* Falls Church, VA: Global Health Solutions, Inc., 1995.

Lawrence, RM, Zucker, M. *Preventing Arthritis.* New York, NY: Berkeley Publishing Group, 2001.

United States Environmental Protection Agency. "Lead and Your Drinking Water." June, 1993.

http://www.yale.edu/ynhti/curriculum/units/1993/5/93.05.06.x.html#j

Vullo-Navich, K, Smith, S, Andrews, M, et al. "Comfort and incidence of abnormal serum sodium, BUN, creatinine and osmolality in dehydration of terminal illness." *American Journal of Hospital Palliative Care.* 15(2):77–84, Mar-Apr 1998.

Chapter 9

Klinkenborg, Verlyn. "Awakening to Sleep." *The New York Times Magazine.* January 5, 1997.

Spiegel, K, Leproult, R, Van Cauter, E. "Impact of sleep debt on metabolic and endocrine function." *The Lancet.* 354(9188):1435–1439, Oct. 23, 1999.

Williamson, AM, Feyer, AM. "Moderate sleep deprivation produces impairments in cognitive and motor performance equivalent to legally prescribed levels of alcohol intoxication." *Occupational and Environmental Medicine.* 57(10):649–655, Oct 2000.

Chapter 10

Brookes, GB. "Vitamin D deficiency and otosclerosis." *Otolaryngology and Head and Neck Surgery.* 93(3):313–321, Jun 1985.

Douglas, WC. *Into The Light.* Miami, FL: Rhino Publishing, 2003. www.rhinopublish.com.

Garland, C, Shekelle, RB, Barrett-Connor, E, et al. "Dietary vitamin D and calcium and risk of colorectal cancer: a 19-year prospective study in men." *The Lancet.* 1(8424):307–309, Feb 9, 1985.

Giovannucci, E, Rimm, EB, Wolk, A, et al."Calcium and fructose intake in relation to risk of prostate cancer." *Cancer Research.* 58(3):442–447, Feb 1, 1998.

Lawson, DE, Paul, AA, Black, AE, et al."Relative contributions of diet and sunlight to vitamin D state in the elderly." *British Journal of Medicine.* 2(6185): 303–305, Aug 4, 1979.

National Research Council. "Diet, Nutrition, and Cancer." Committee on Diet, Nutrition, and Cancer, Assembly of Life Sciences, National Research Council, National Academy Press, Washington, D.C., 1982.

Chapter 11

Basu, TK. "High-dose ascorbic acid decreases detoxification of cyanide derived from amygdalin (laetrile): studies in guinea pigs." *Canadian Journal of Physiology and Pharmacology.* 61(11):1426–1430, Nov 1983.

Cadenas, S, Rojas, C, Perez-Campo, R, et al. "Vitamin E protects guinea pig liver from lipid peroxidation without depressing levels of antioxidants." *International al Journal of Biochemical Cell Biology.* 27(11):1175–1181, Nov 1995.

Krishnamurthy, S, George, T, Jayanthi Bai, N. "Effect of dietary coconut oil and casein and megadoses of vitamin A or C on tissue lipid peroxidation and hemolysis in vitamin E deficiency." *Acta Vitaminologica et Enzymologica.* 5(3):165–170, 1983.

Chapter 12

Boissonneault, GA, Elson, CE, Pariza, MW. "Net energy effects of dietary fat on chemically induced mammary carcinogenesis in F344 rats." *Journal of the National Cancer Institute.* 76(2):335–338, Feb 1986.

Duran, M, Loof, NE, Ketting, et al. "Secondary carnitine deficiency." *Journal of Clinical Chemistry and Clinical Biochemistry.* 28(5):359–363, May 1990.

Etzioni, A, Levy, J, Nitzan, M, et al. "Systemic carnitine deficiency exacerbated by a strict vegetarian diet." *Archives of Disease in Childhood.* 59(2):177–179, Feb 1984.

Flachs, P, Horakova, O, Brauner, P, et al. "Polyunsaturated fatty acids of marine origin upregulate mitochondrial biogenesis and induce beta-oxidation in white fat." *Diabetologia.* 48(11):2365–2375, Nov 2005. Epub Oct 5, 2005.

Holmes, MD, Hunter, DJ, et al. "Association of Dietary Intake of Fat and Fatty Acids With Risk of Breast Cancer." *Journal of the American Medical Association (JAMA)* 281:914–920, 1999.

Ide, T, Watanabe, M, Sugano, M, et al. "Activities of liver mitochondrial and peroxisomal fatty acid oxidation enzymes in rats fed trans fat." *Lipids.* 22(1):6–10, Jan 1987.

Larque, E, Garcia-Ruiz, PA, Perez-Llamas, F, et al. "Dietary trans fatty acids alter the compositions of microsomes and mitochondria and the activities of microsome delta6-fatty acid desaturase and glucose-6-phosphatase in livers of pregnant rats." *The Journal of Nutrition.* 133(8):2526–2531, Aug 2003.

Lombard, KA, Olson, AL, Nelson, SE, et al. "Carnitine status of lactoovovegetarians and strict vegetarian adults and children." *American Journal of Clinical Nutrition.* 50(2):301–306, Aug 1989.

Majchrzak, D, Singer, I, Manner, M, et al. "B-Vitamin Status and Concentrations of Homocysteine in Austrian Omnivores, Vegetarians and Vegans." *Annals of Nutritional Metabolism.* 50(6):485–491, Sep 19, 2006.

Roberts, Michelle. "Children 'harmed' by vegan diets." BBC News health reporter, in Washington DC. Feb 21, 2005.

Spiller, G, Spiller, M. *What's with Fiber.* Laguna Beach, CA: Basic Health Publications, 2005.

Chapter 13

Arkin, SM, "Student-led exercise sessions yield significant fitness gains for Alzheimer's patient." *American Journal of Alzheimer's Disease and Other Dementias.* 18(3):159–170, 2003.

Babyak, M, Blumenthal, JA, Herman, S, et al. "Exercise treatment for major depression: maintenance of therapeutic benefit at 10 months." *Psychosomatic Medicine.* 62(5):633–638, Sep-Oct 2000.

Blair, SN, Kohl, HW, Paffenbarger, RS, et al. "Physical fitness and all cause mortality. A prospective study of healthy men and women." *Journal of the American Medical Association (JAMA).* 262(17):2395-401, Nov 3, 1989.

Larson, EB, Wang, L, Bowen, JD, et al. "Exercise is associated with reduced risk for incident dementia among persons 65 years of age and older." *Annals of Internal Medicine.* 144(2):73–81, Jan 17, 2006.

Laukkanen, JA, Lakka, TA, Rauramaa, R, et al. "Cardiovascular fitness as a predictor of mortality in men." *Archives of Internal Medicine.* 161(6):825–831, Mar 26, 2001.

Nelson, R. "Exercise could prevent cerebral changes associated with AD." *Lancet Neurology.* 4(5):275, May 2005.

Paffenbarger, RS, Hyde, RT, Wing, AL, et al. "Physical activity, all cause mortality, and longevity of college alumni." *New England Journal of Medicine.* 314(10):605–613, Mar 6, 1986.

Pahor, M, Guralnik, JM, Salive, ME, et al. "Physical activity and risk of severe gastrointestinal hemorrhage in older persons." *Journal of the American Medical Association (JAMA).* 272(8):595–599, Aug 24–31, 1994.

Pinnock, CB, Stapleton, AM, Marshall, VR. "Erectile dysfunction in the community: a prevalence study." *Medical Journal of Australia.* 171:353–357, 1999.

Chapter 15

Barnes, B. *Hypothyroidism, The Unsuspected Illness.* New York, NY: HarperCollins, 1976.

Blask, DE, Brainard, GC, et al. "Melatonin-depleted blood from premenopausal women exposed to light at night stimulates growth of human breast cancer xenografts in nude rats." *Cancer Research.* 65:11174–11184. Dec 1, 2005.

Carruthers, Malcolm. *Maximizing Manhood: How to Beat the Male Menopause.* London, England: Thorsons; New Ed edition, 1998.

Ettinger, B, Friedman, GD, Bush, T, et al. "Reduced mortality associated with long-term postmenopausal estrogen therapy." *Obstetrics and Gynecology.* 87(1):6–12, Jan 1996.

Garfinkel, D, Laudon, M, Nof, D, et al. "Improvement of sleep quality in elderly people by controlled-release melatonin." *The Lancet.* 346(8974):541–544, Aug 26, 1995.

Gower, BA, Nyman, L. "Associations among Oral Estrogen Use, Free Testosterone Concentration, and Lean Body Mass among Postmenopausal Women." *The Journal of Clinical Endocrinology and Metabolism.* 85(12):4476–4480, Dec 2000.

Henderson, BE, Paganini-Hill, A, Ross, RK. "Decreased mortality in users of estrogen replacement therapy." *Archives of Internal Medicine.* 151(1):75–78, Jan 1991.

Lissoni, P; Barni, S; Meregalli, S; et al. "Modulation of cancer endocrine therapy by melatonin: a phase II study of tamoxifen plus melatonin in metastatic breast cancer patients progressing under tamoxifen alone." *British Journal of Cancer (ENGLAND).* 71(4):854–856, Apr 1995.

Ly, LP, Jimenez, M, Zhuang, TN, et al. "A double-blind, placebo-controlled, randomized clinical trial of transdermal dihydrotestosterone gel on muscular strength, mobility, and quality of life in older men with partial androgen deficiency." *The Journal of Clinical Endocrinology and Metabolism.* 86(9):4078–4088, Sep 2001.

Maestroni, GJ. "The immunoneuroendocrine role of melatonin." *Journal of Pineal Research.* 14(1):1–10, Jan 1993.

Marin, P, Holmang, S, Jonsson, L, et al. "The effects of testosterone treatment on body composition and metabolism in middle-aged obese men." *International Journal of Obesity Related Metabolic Disorders.* 16(12):991–997, Dec 1992.

Moretti, RM, Marelli, MM, Maggi, R, et al. "Antiproliferative action of melatonin on human prostate cancer LNCaP cells." *Oncology Reports.* 7(2):347–351, 2000.

Page, ST, Amory, JK, Bowman, FD, et al. "Exogenous testosterone (T) alone or with finasteride increases physical performance, grip strength, and lean body mass in older men with low serum T." *Journal of Clinical Endocrinology Metabolism.* 90(3):1502–1510, Mar 2005.

Pierpaoli, W, Lesnikov, V. "Pineal cross-transplantation (old-to-young and vice versa) as evidence for an endogenous 'aging clock'." *Annals of the New York Academy of Sciences.* 719:456–460, May 31, 1994.

Pierpaoli, W, Regelson, W. *The Melatonin Miracle: Nature's Age-Reversing, Disease-Fighting, Sex-Enhancing Hormone.* New York, NY: Pocket Books div of Simon and Schuster, 1995.

Reiss, U, Zucker, M. *Natural Hormone Balance for Women: Look Younger, Feel Stronger, and Live Life with Exuberance.* New York, NY: Simon and Shuster, 1996.

Rudman, D, Feller, AG, Cohn, L, et al. "Effects of human growth hormone on body composition in elderly men." *Hormone Research.* 36 Suppl 1:73–81, 1991.

Rudman, D, Feller, AG, Nagraj, HS, et al." Effects of human growth hormone in men over 60 years old." *New England Journal of Medicine.* 323(1):1–6, Jul 5, 1990.

Sahelian, R. *Melatonin: Nature's Sleeping Pill.* 2nd ed. London, England: Avery Publishing, The Penguin Group, 1996.

Savine, R, Sonksen, P. "Growth hormone - hormone replacement for the somatopause?" *Hormone Research.* 53 Suppl 3:37–41, 2000.

Schernhammer, ES, Hankinson, SE. "Urinary melatonin levels and breast cancer risk." *Journal of the National Cancer Institute.* 97:1084–1087, July 20, 2005.

Tan, DX, Reiter, RJ, Manchester, LC, et al. "Chemical and physical properties and potential mechanisms: melatonin as a broad spectrum antioxidant and free radical scavenger." *Current Topics in Medcine and Chemistry.* 2(2):181–197, Feb 2002.

Valenta, LJ, Elias, AN."How to detect hypothyroidism when screening tests are normal. Use of the TRH stimulation test," Postgraduate Medicine. 72(2):267–274, Aug 1983.

Van Cauter, E, Leproult, R, Plat, L. "Age-related changes in slow wave sleep and REM sleep and relationship with growth hormone and cortisol levels in healthy men." *Journal of the American Medical Association (JAMA)* 340. 284(7):861–868, Aug 16, 2000.

Verkasalo, PK, Stevens, RG, et al. "Sleep duration and breast cancer: A prospective cohort study." *Cancer Research.* 65:9595–9600, Oct 15, 2005.

Index

About the Author

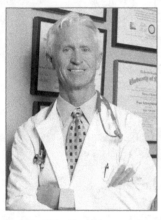

Frank Shallenberger, M.D., has devoted his professional career to understanding the fundamentals of what keeps people well. To this end, he has, for more than twenty years, used an approach in his medical practice that integrates the best of alternative medicine with the best of conventional medicine.

He is a pioneer in the clinical application of oxidative medicine, a new discipline that emphasizes the profound importance of oxygen and energy production in health and longevity.

Dr. Shallenberger is the founder and medical director of The Nevada Center of Alternative and Anti-Aging Medicine in Carson City, Nevada, a facility that attracts people from all over the country. He is board-certified in Anti-Aging Medicine, and has served as a clinical instructor in Family Medicine at the University of California School of Medicine in Davis. In 2001, he was honored to be a speaker in Monte Carlo at the First International Learning Conference on Anti-Aging Medicine, a global gathering of health professionals interested in applying anti-aging strategies.

Shallenberger is the father of four children, and grandfather to three. His extended family includes a horse, two llamas, a dog, five sheep, and ten chickens. An avid backpacker and cyclist, he has won numerous cycling events, and garnered silver medals in the Nevada State Mountain Bike Championship Series and the Northern California Time Trials. He aims to keep himself and his patients young and energetic for a long, long time.